Feed Your Mind - How Does Nutrition Modulate Brain Function throughout Life?

Edited by Clémentine Bosch-Bouju, Sophie Layé and Véronique Pallet

Published in London, United Kingdom

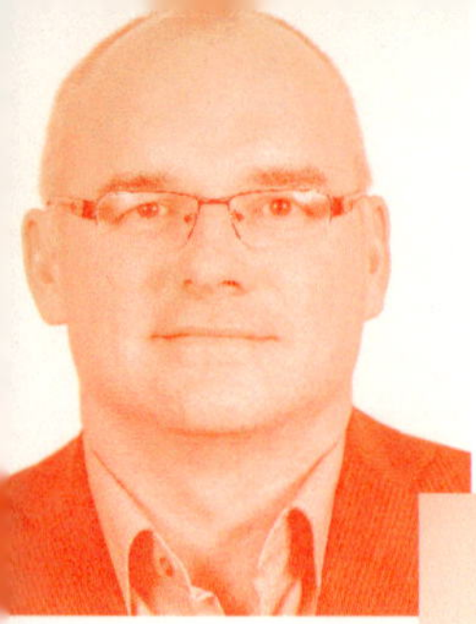
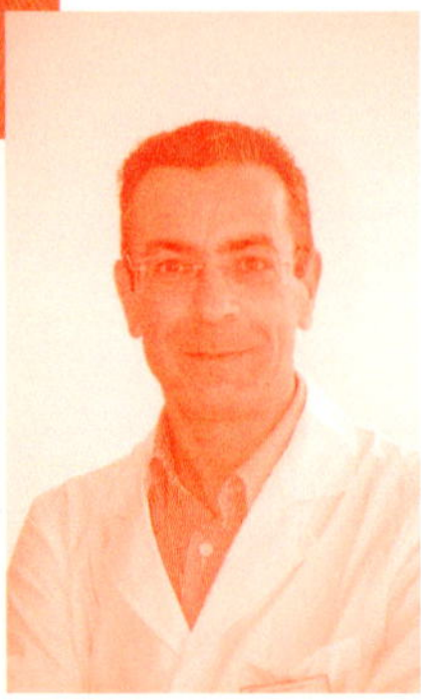
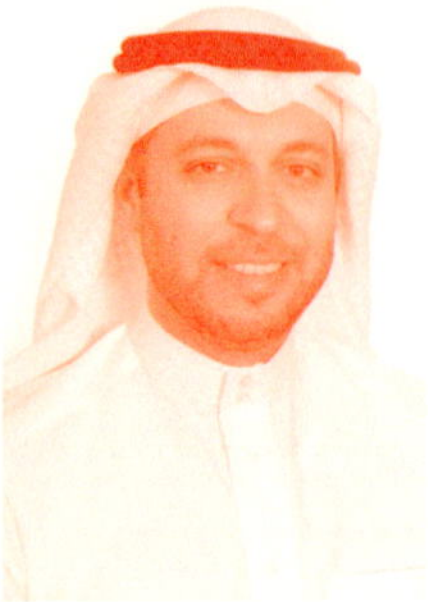
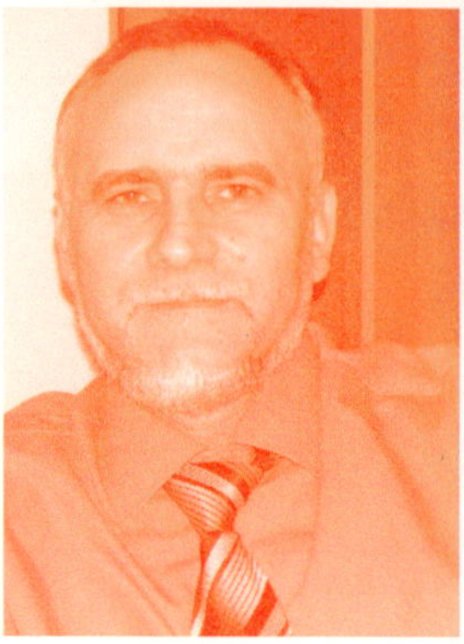
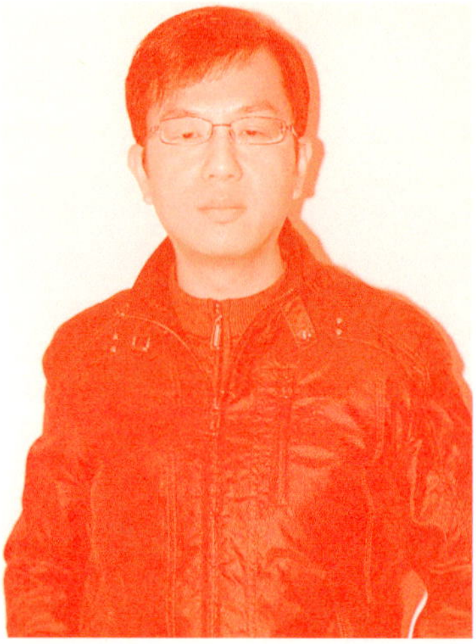
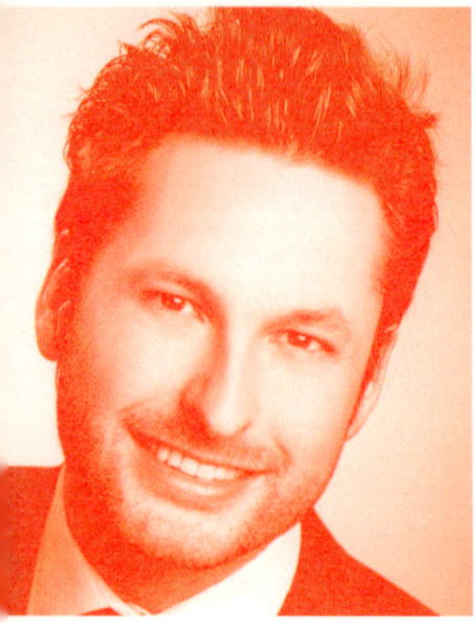
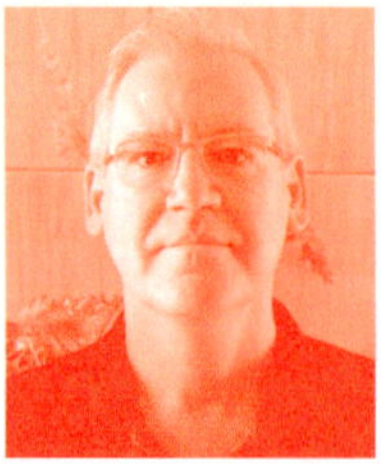

IntechOpen

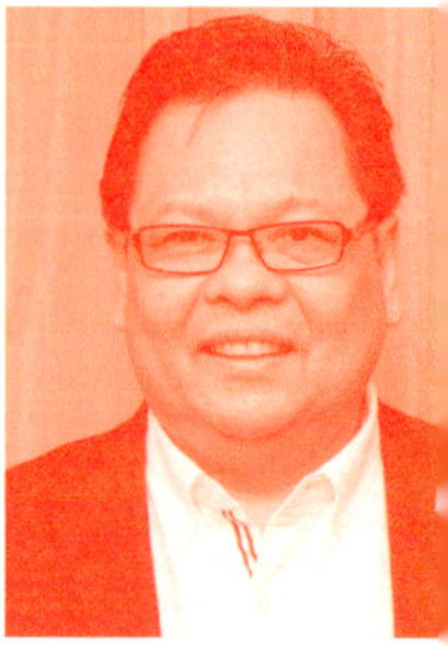
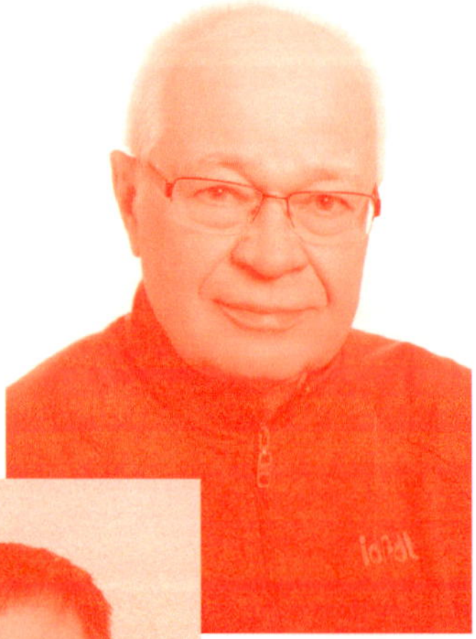
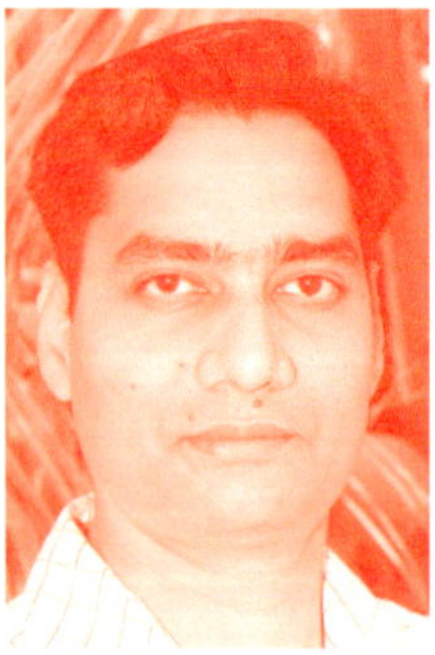
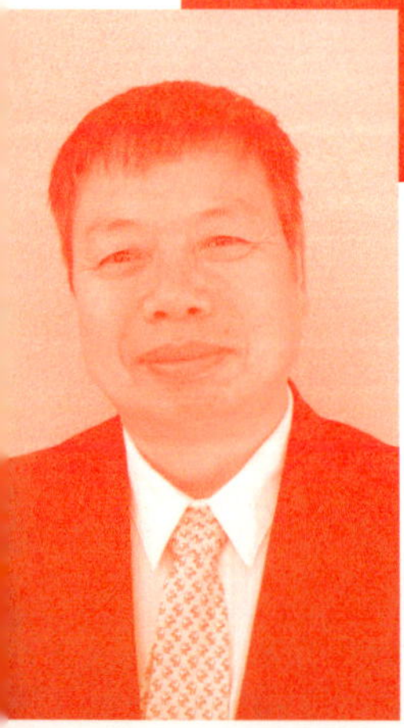
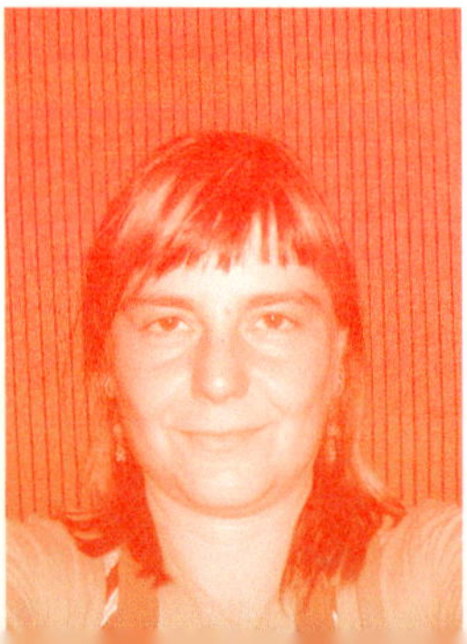
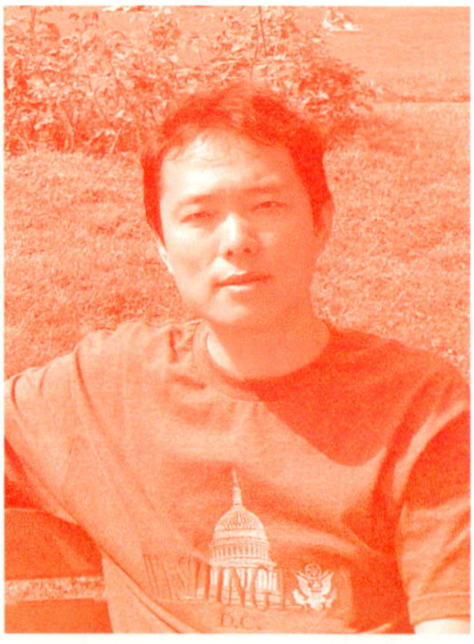

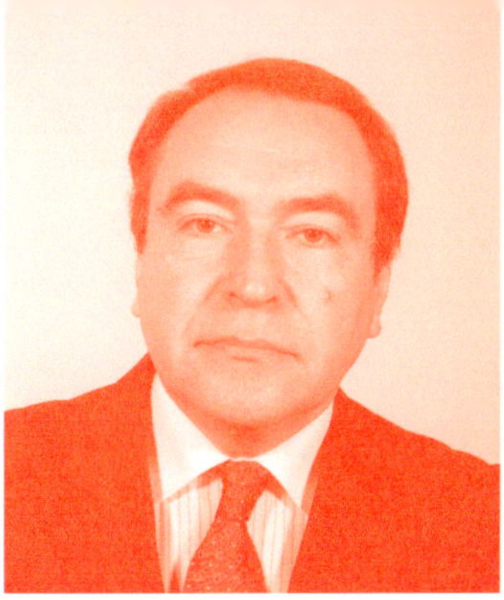
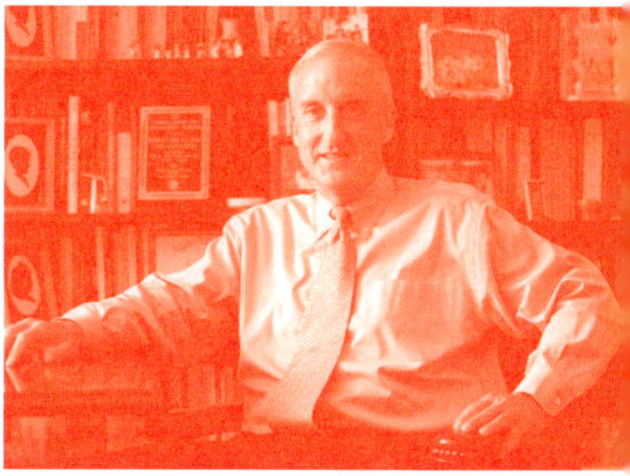
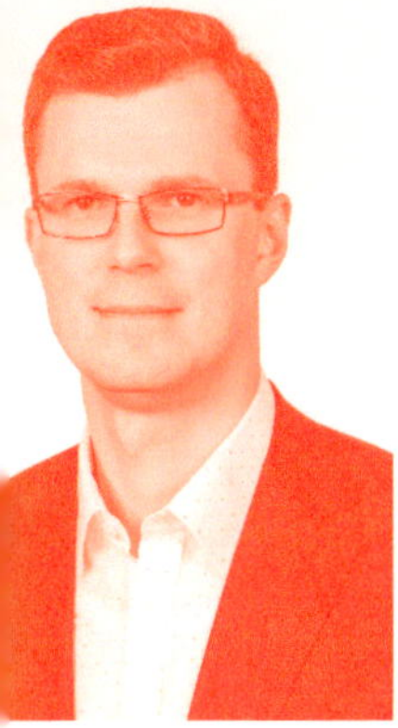
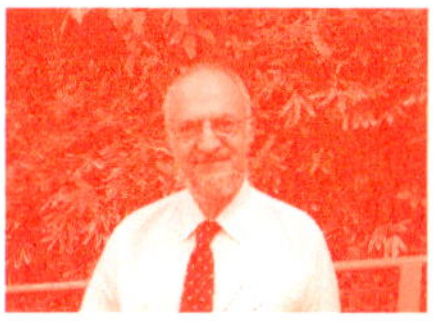
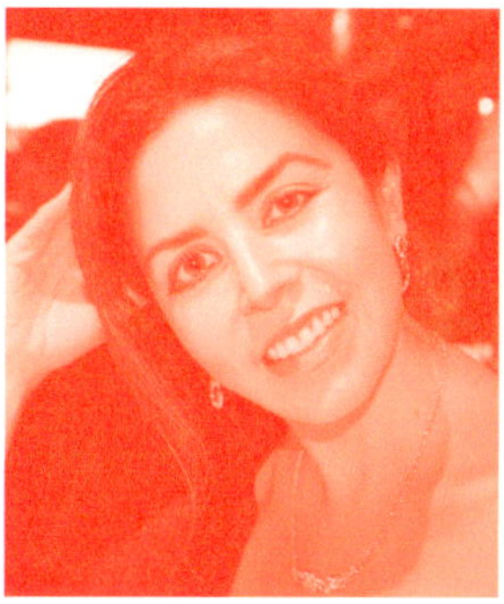

Supporting open minds since 2005

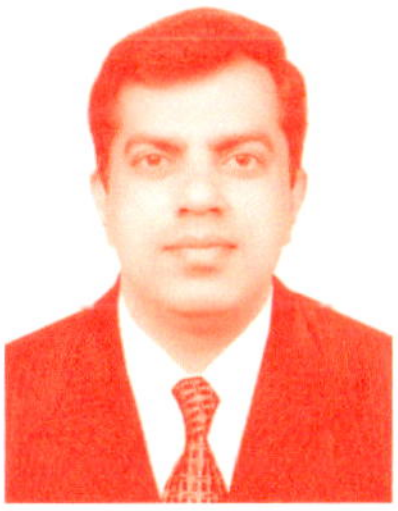
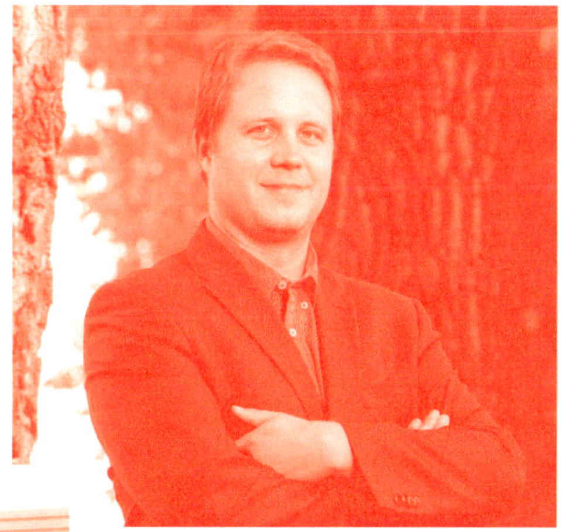
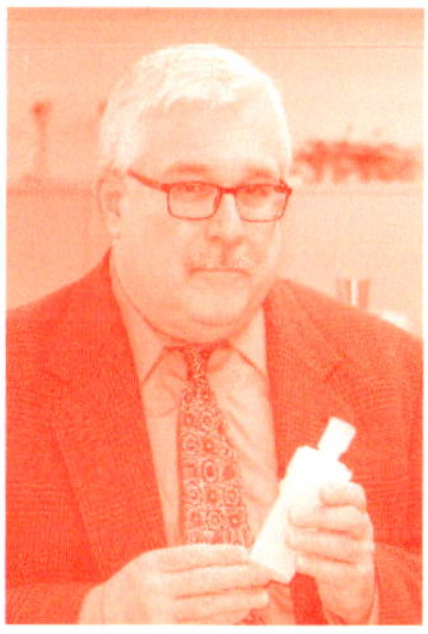
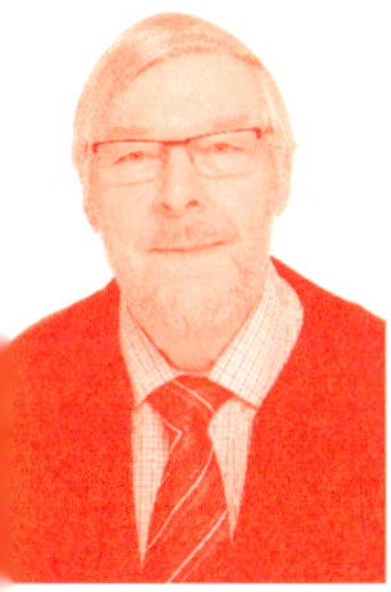
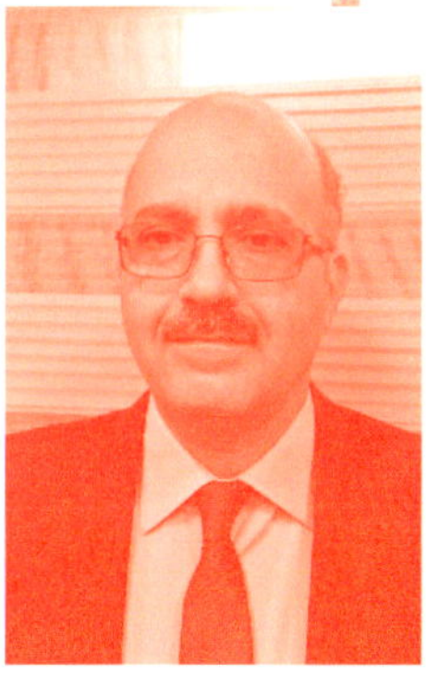
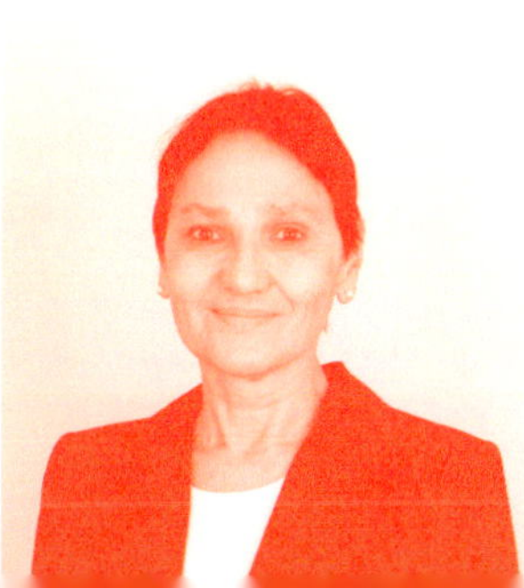
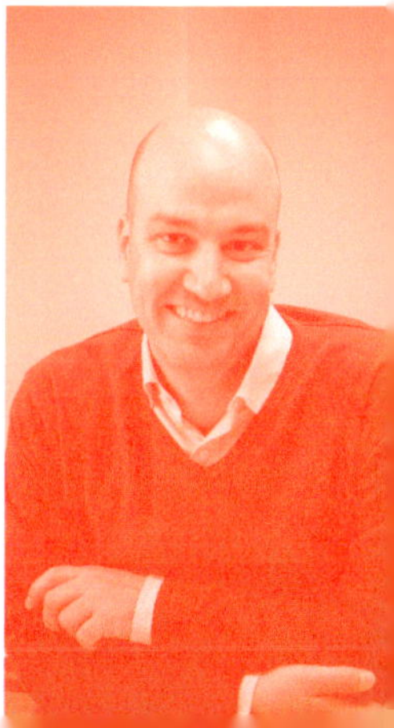

Feed Your Mind - How Does Nutrition Modulate Brain Function throughout Life?
http://dx.doi.org/10.5772/intechopen.73436
Edited by Clémentine Bosch-Bouju, Sophie Layé and Véronique Pallet

Contributors
Javier Mahía, María Ángeles Zafra Palma, Amadeo Puerto, María J. Simón, Filomena Molina, Ben Loos, Claudia Ntsapi, Andre du Toit, Corinne Joffre, Xavier Fioramonti, Luc Pénicaud, Clémentine Bosch-Bouju

First published in London, United Kingdom, 2019 by IntechOpen
IntechOpen is the global imprint of INTECHOPEN LIMITED, registered in England and Wales, registration number: 11086078, The Shard, 25th floor, 32 London Bridge Street
London, SE19SG - United Kingdom
Printed in Croatia

British Library Cataloguing-in-Publication Data
A catalogue record for this book is available from the British Library

Additional hard and PDF copies can be obtained from orders@intechopen.com

Feed Your Mind - How Does Nutrition Modulate Brain Function throughout Life?
Edited by Clémentine Bosch-Bouju, Sophie Layé and Véronique Pallet
p. cm.
Print ISBN 978-1-78985-582-1
Online ISBN 978-1-83962-511-4
eBook (PDF) ISBN 978-1-83962-512-1

Meet the editors

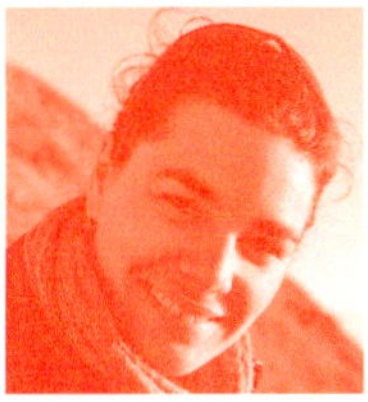

Dr. Clémentine Bosch-Bouju is a neuroscientist expert in the impact of nutrition on neurophysiology. She did her PhD in the Collège De France, Paris, and her postdoc at the University of Otago, New Zealand, on the physiopathology of Parkinson's disease, with electrophysiology and optogenetics approaches. She joined the NutriNeuro lab in 2014 where she specialized in the impact of nutrition on brain function. Her work shows the deleterious impact of an omega-3-deficient diet on endocannabinoid-dependent synaptic plasticity. Since 2016, Dr. Bosch-Bouju has been an assistant professor at Bordeaux INP and she is studying the role of vitamin A metabolism in the pathophysiology of Parkinson's disease.

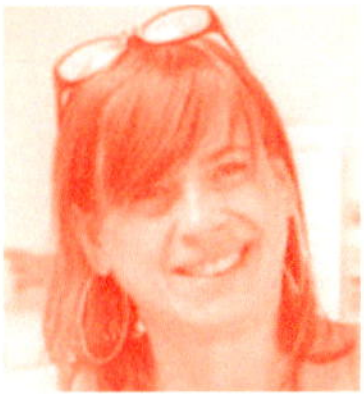

Sophie Layé, PhD, is a research director at the Institut National de la Recherche en Agronomie (INRA), France. She is the acting head of the NutriNeuro Institute (UMR1286 INRA/University of Bordeaux) and co-acting head of the International Associated Laboratory OptiNutriBrain. She is a renowned scientist in the field of psychoneuroimmunology. She was the first to demonstrate that dietary omega-3 impacts on the endocannabinoid system to modulate emotional behaviors. She has authored more than 105 original scientific articles and 14 book chapters. She is reviewer for more than 15 international scientific journals. She has organized more than 30 international congresses and conferences, given more than 110 conferences, and participated in more than 80 press releases in the media. She received the prestigious Scientific Breakthrough Award, Laurier de l'INRA, in 2015.

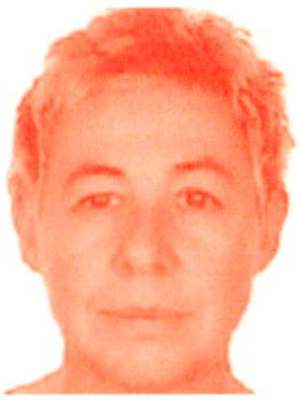

Véronique Pallet, PhD, is a professor at the Bordeaux Institute of Technology and co-head of the NutriNeuro Institute (UMR1286 INRA/University of Bordeaux). She is a renowned scientist in the field of nutrition and its impact on age-related cognitive decline and neurodegenerative processes. She is recognized in the field of vitamin A and cognition, and her team has demonstrated the role of this liposoluble vitamin in maintaining cognitive abilities during aging. She is also investigating the role of polyphenol in memory processes in the Neurophenols Project. She recently conducted two clinical trials, conducted in France and Québec, investigating the beneficial impact of nutritional supplementations on cognitive abilities and well-being assessed in aged subjects. She has authored more than 60 scientific articles and reviews in high-impact journals.

Contents

Preface

Modern societies have recently experienced several transitions in dietary habits. The last few centuries have emerged from famine by increasing the consumption of cereals. Also, food production has been industrialized, which enhances the diversity of food products. However, food industrialization also induces a rise in saturated fats and sugars in the diet, paralleled by a reduction in physical activity. More developed countries are now in a new transition phase fueled by the desire for healthier and less processed food. With these dietary transitions, human health has evolved, following the famous adage "We are what we eat." The most obvious example is the important escalation in diabetes occurrence over the last 30 years or so. Therefore, nutrition is a critical environmental factor modulating health throughout life.

Over the past decades, scientific interest has been focused on the impact of nutrition specifically on brain function. Several years of research have established that nutrients such as polyunsaturated fatty acids, vitamins, polyphenols, essential amino acids, and sugar are the basis for brain function and their imbalance can cause or precipitate brain dysfunction.

Most nutrients can cross the blood–brain barrier to impact brain physiology. Nutrients in the brain can either fuel brain cells, contribute to tissue architecture, or initiate signaling pathways through their derivatives. Nutrients ultimately participate in brain development, cognitive and emotional behaviors, and can influence the susceptibility to develop brain pathologies. Despite the huge amount of knowledge brought about by the scientific community, a lot still needs to be unraveled.

Beyond dietary habits, nutrients can also be isolated and formulated to serve as therapeutic agents. Indeed, they are less prone to develop secondary effects than pharmaceuticals since the organism has the machinery to metabolize them. In addition, they can enter the brain more easily than synthetic molecules, which is essential to reach therapeutic efficacy for brain-related disorders.

More recently, the field of brain nutrition has been enlarged by considering bidirectional interactions between the brain and the periphery, including microbiota and the enteric system. For example, some microbiota species release derivatives following digestion and can have a direct effect on brain function. In the other direction, it is now clear that the brain can control digestion and metabolism, not only through the hypothalamus, but also through mechanisms and circuits that are highly sophisticated, which delay their precise understanding. In addition, these bidirectional interactions between the brain and the periphery for nutrition are interdependent, which further complicates the picture.

Feed Your Mind: How Does Nutrition Modulate Brain Function throughout Life? is a selection of current research on the impact of diet on brain function. The book is organized into five chapters, opening with the editor's Introductory chapter.

Chapter 2 is dedicated to the role of lipids in the brain. In particular, polyunsaturated fatty acids are highly enriched in the brain and brain cells. This chapter focuses on these polyunsaturated fatty acids and their derivatives, involved in the resolution of neuroinflammation.

Chapter 3 focuses on the role of glucose in fueling the brain, and how some hypothalamic neurons are sensitive to glycemia, to participate in its regulation. Indeed, the brain represents approximately 2% of body weight but consumes approximately 20% of its total energy. Therefore, blood glucose is essential for brain function. This chapter also discusses the role of fructose in brain function, since the current industrialized diet contains abnormally high levels of fructose.

Chapter 4 presents the concept of autophagy and how nutrition can modulate it. Autophagy is a process of protein degradation in cells that allow control of cell integrity. Autophagy is stimulated by caloric restriction; however, the global trend in industrialized countries is toward calories over consumption. Therefore, this chapter presents how modern dietary habits can favor neuropathologies associated with autophagy defects, such as in Alzheimer's disease.

Finally, Chapter 5 concentrates on brain–gut interactions in the context of enteral feeding. Some chronic pathologies require non-oral feeding, which basically bypasses the brain in the control of feeding. This particular situation highlights the role of the brain in different steps of feeding, from appetite to digestion. This chapter also points out strategies to improve digestion in enteral feeding.

We would like to thank all the authors for their valuable contributions and for their constructive interplay throughout the editorial process.

Clémentine Bosch-Bouju, Sophie Layé and Véronique Pallet
NutriNeuro Lab UMR1286,
INRA/Bordeaux University/Bordeaux INP,
France

Section 1

Introduction

Chapter 1

Introductory Chapter: Feed Your Mind - How Does Nutrition Modulate Brain Function throughout Life?

Clémentine Bosch-Bouju

1. Introduction

Nutrition is a transdisciplinary science that aims at studying the role of food and physical exercise on health and diseases. It includes notably biochemistry, metabolism, behavioural and social studies. Nutrition science is highly diverse and constantly evolving for several reasons:

- The control of energy balance is a primary need for humans and for all animals, which implies it is of high importance.
- A high diversity of dietary models throughout the world exists, which is closely related to the diversity of culture, even in one single country.
- In human societies, alimentation participates to social behaviour.
- Modern societies have been hugely transformed since food industrialization.

The last point has critically changed the way of life for people in industrialised countries. Food industrialisation was originally designed to ease life and feed the growing population following the First and Second World Wars. Unexpectedly, industrialisation has engendered a profound dietary imbalance.

For the first time in history, people with industrialised diet are facing food with high quantities of sugar and saturated fats. This diet can also lead to deficiency in essential nutrients, such as vitamins, minerals and polyunsaturated fatty acids. This change in diet has been paralleled by an increase in sedentariness, which contributes to energy imbalance. This change in the last 70 years leads to global epidemics as obesity, cardiovascular disorders and depressive disorders.

In this context, the brain appears as a structure highly sensitive to dietary imbalance [1]. In addition, the brain can participate to dietary imbalance by controlling feeding behaviours and through its interaction with peripheral organs and hormones involved in the control of energy balance. Thus, the impact of nutrition on brain function is a specific field of research that has gain interest in the recent years, and the role of the brain appears central in nutrition. Nutrition will impact the brain from early-developmental stages to adolescence, when the brain tissue is built and modelled. Nutrition also appears critical at adult age, to maintain optimal brain function. Finally, nutrition appears as an important environmental factor that

IntechOpen

should be controlled through ageing, to prevent neurodegenerative processes. In this introductory chapter, we will take the example of vitamin A, which is a nutrient that has been demonstrated as critical for brain function throughout life [2–5].

2. Vitamin A and its active metabolite: retinoic acid

Vitamin A is a lipophilic vitamin that cannot be synthesised de novo by organism. Food sources are animal products for the preformed vitamin A and vegetables for provitamin A. Preformed vitamin A and provitamin A are found in sufficient quantities in most diets, but strong deficiency may occur in undernourished populations, mainly in sub-Saharan Africa. Vitamin A deficiency in children can cause blindness and growth retardation and can ultimately lead to death. Besides, vitamin A deficiency may occur with ageing, since its bioavailability can be reduced. In both cases, vitamin A supplementation can reverse this deficiency, which emphasises the need to study the impact of vitamin A supplementation for pregnant women and children, as well as for elderly.

The active metabolite of vitamin A in the brain is the all-*trans* retinoic acid (a*t*RA), synthesised from vitamin A (retinol) by aldehyde dehydrogenase enzymes [6, 7]. Retinoic acid and its derivatives bind to nuclear receptors, namely, RAR and RXR. These receptors act as homo- or heterodimers to control gene transcription [3, 6]. Therefore, retinoic acid is a powerful morphogen factor, highly involved in embryonic development and growth [8].

3. The role of vitamin A during brain development

During brain development, retinoic acid synthesised from dietary vitamin A binds to nuclear receptors to drive transcription of hundreds of genes. Retinoic acid is a morphogen that acts through a concentration gradient [8]. To carry out the precision of retinoic acid gradient during embryonic development, metabolism and signalling pathways for retinoic acid are multiple and highly robust [8]. Remarkably, retinoic acid is the only morphogen that comes from dietary sources, which highlights the importance of vitamin A intake during pregnancy. Through its action on nuclear receptors, retinoic acid is implicated in the patterning of neural axis along the dorsoventral and anteroposterior axes [2].

In addition to development and growth, retinoic acid in the brain is critical for neuronal differentiation and neurite outgrowth. This is particularly true in the basal ganglia network, which is a group of brain structures involved in the control of action. Indeed, retinoic acid is key in the differentiation of specific subpopulations of neurons, such as the medium size spiny neurons in the striatum, or the dopaminergic neurons from the substantia nigra pars compacta [9–13].

4. The role of vitamin A in the adult brain

At adult age, vitamin A-derived retinoic acid has two remarkable roles; it is involved in homeostatic plasticity and in neurogenesis [3, 5, 14, 15]. First, retinoic acid induces molecular and morphological changes in neuronal network, to maintain overall synaptic activity constant, despite synaptic plasticity, a process named homeostatic synaptic plasticity [16]. For this, retinoic acid binds to nuclear RAR and RXR receptors, but evidence suggests that non-genomic mechanisms are also involved [17–19]. Changes induced by retinoic acid to produce homeostatic plasticity include transcription of synaptic proteins, such as AMPA receptors, but also modulation of neuronal morphology, through outgrowth or retraction of synapse boutons and dendrites.

Second, retinoic acid controls neurogenesis. In rodent deficient for vitamin A, neurogenesis in the hippocampus is strongly dampened and can be restored by replenishment with vitamin A or derivatives [20–23]. However, in physiological conditions, retinoic acid applied exogenously can inhibit neurogenesis in the hippocampus and facilitate cell differentiation [3]. The apparent discrepancy between physiological and deficient states may be explained by the finely tuned concentration and timing of retinoic acid that is needed for its control of neurogenesis. In the hypothalamus, neurogenesis is highly dynamic to orchestrate circadian rhythms that govern several hypothalamic functions. In this structure, a similar role has been demonstrated for retinoic acid, inhibiting proliferation of cells and thus neurogenesis [5].

5. The role of vitamin A in the ageing brain

Ageing process is a physiological and unavoidable phenomenon involving the whole body. Related to brain function, ageing is characterised by a cognitive decline, which comprises all molecular and cellular alterations that lead ultimately to decreased performance in cognitive and executive functions [24]. Evidence suggests that bioavailability of retinoic acid in the brain reduces with ageing, likely due to peripheral alterations [4]. Yet several studies have highlighted the parallel between ageing, decrease in brain retinoid signalling and cognitive decline [4, 25–27]. Mechanisms linking retinoid metabolism and cognitive decline are not yet completely unravelled, but evidence suggests the involvement of glucocorticoids [20] and morphological changes of neuronal trees (unpublished data).

Beyond normal ageing, decreased retinoid signalling in the brain with ageing may be involved in neurodegenerative processes, such as in Alzheimer's and Parkinson's diseases. For Alzheimer's disease, accumulating evidence suggests that the lack of retinoic acid in the hippocampus is a risk factor that precipitates the deposition of β-amyloid plaques, a histological landmark of the disease [28–31]. Therefore, vitamin A and retinoids appear as potential therapeutics [30, 32]. However, mechanisms are not yet sufficiently understood to elaborate such therapeutics. Additionally, retinoids are lipophilic molecules that oxidise rapidly, which render their pharmacological use challenging.

In the context of Parkinson's disease, a similar process has been proposed. Reduced signalling of retinoids in the brain, and particularly in the substantia nigra compacta, may be a risk factor that accelerates the degeneration of dopaminergic neurons [33, 34]. This hypothesis is supported by the fact that rodents deficient for vitamin A or for retinoid receptors display motor impairments close to Parkinson's models [35, 36]. Some studies revealed encouraging results with retinoid supplementation to prevent neurodegeneration in cell culture or in vivo [37, 38], but research is still to preliminary to envisage soon vitamin A-based treatments for this disease.

6. Conclusion

Through the solely example of vitamin A, we can appreciate the importance of nutrition for brain physiology, from development to adult age. Remarkably, a same nutrient can have different roles depending on the timing, the brain structure and even the cell type. The field of research on nutrition applied to neurosciences is growing, to better encompass the impact of industrialised diet on brain function and also to consider nutrients and their derivatives as potential therapeutic strategies. In this way, it is to expect that nutritional approaches will give rise in the future to new therapeutics to prevent, and in some case cure, neurological disorders.

Author details

Clémentine Bosch-Bouju
INRA, Bordeaux INP, NutriNeuro, University of Bordeaux, Bordeaux, France

*Address all correspondence to: clementine.bosch-bouju@inra.fr

References

[1] Gómez-Pinilla F. Brain foods: The effects of nutrients on brain function. Nature Reviews. Neuroscience. 2008;**9**(7):568-578

[2] Maden M. Retinoic acid in the development, regeneration and maintenance of the nervous system. Nature Reviews. Neuroscience. 2007;**8**(10):755-765

[3] McCaffery P, Zhang J, Crandall JE. Retinoic acid signaling and function in the adult hippocampus. Journal of Neurobiology. 2006;**66**(7):780-791

[4] Sauvant P,Feart C, Sauvant J, Pallet V. Vitamin A and cognitive impairment. In: Diet and Nutrition in Dementia and Cognitive Decline. Advances in Clinical Neuroscience and Rehabilitation; 2015. pp. 623-635. Available from: https://linkinghub.elsevier.com/retrieve/pii/B9780124078246000586

[5] Shearer KD, Stoney PN, Morgan PJ, McCaffery PJ. A vitamin for the brain. Trends in Neurosciences. 2012;**35**(12):733-741

[6] Blomhoff R, Blomhoff HK. Overview of retinoid metabolism and function. Journal of Neurobiology. 2006;**66**(7):606-630

[7] Koppaka V, Thompson DC, Chen Y, Ellermann M, Nicolaou KC, Juvonen RO, et al. Aldehyde dehydrogenase inhibitors: A comprehensive review of the pharmacology, mechanism of action, substrate specificity, and clinical application. The American Society for Pharmacology and Experimental Therapeutics. Pharmacological Reviews. 2012;**64**(3):520-539

[8] Schilling TF, Nie Q, Lander AD. Dynamics and precision in retinoic acid morphogen gradients. Current Opinion in Genetics and Development. 2012;**22**(6):562-569

[9] Chatzi C, Brade T, Duester G. Retinoic acid functions as a key GABAergic differentiation signal in the basal ganglia. PLoS Biology. 2011;**9**(4):e1000609

[10] Occhi G, Regazzo D, Albiger NM, Ceccato F, Ferasin S, Scanarini M, et al. Activation of the dopamine receptor Type-2 (DRD2) promoter by 9-cis retinoic acid in a cellular model of Cushing's disease mediates the inhibition of cell proliferation and ACTH secretion without a complete corticotroph-to-melanotroph transdifferentiation. Endocrinology. 2014;**155**(9):3538-3549

[11] Pedrini S, Bogush A, Ehrlich ME. Phosphatidylinositide 3-kinase and protein kinase C zeta mediate retinoic acid induction of DARPP-32 in medium size spiny neurons in vitro. Journal of Neurochemistry. 2008;**106**(2):917-924

[12] Podleśny-Drabiniok A, Sobska J, de Lera AR, Gołembiowska K, Kamińska K, Dollé P, et al. Distinct retinoic acid receptor (RAR) isotypes control differentiation of embryonal carcinoma cells to dopaminergic or striatopallidal medium spiny neurons. Scientific Reports. 2017;**7**(1):13671

[13] Rataj-Baniowska M, Niewiadomska-Cimicka A, Paschaki M, Szyszka-Niagolov M, Carramolino L, Torres M, et al. Retinoic acid receptor β controls development of Striatonigral projection neurons through FGF-dependent and Meis1-dependent mechanisms. Journal of Neuroscience: The Official Journal of the Society for Neuroscience. 2015;**35**(43):14467-14475

[14] Lane MA, Bailey SJ. Role of retinoid signalling in the adult brain. Progress in Neurobiology. 2005;**75**(4):275-293

[15] Olson CR, Mello CV. Significance of vitamin A to brain function, behavior and learning. Molecular Nutrition and Food Research. 2010;**54**(4):489-495

[16] Turrigiano GG, Nelson SB. Homeostatic plasticity in the developing nervous system. Nature Reviews. Neuroscience. 2004;**5**(2):97-107

[17] Aoto J, Nam CI, Poon MM, Ting P, Chen L. Synaptic signaling by all-trans retinoic acid in homeostatic synaptic plasticity. Neuron. 2008;**60**(2):308-320

[18] Arendt KL, Zhang Y, Jurado S, Malenka RC, Südhof TC, Chen L. Retinoic acid and LTP recruit postsynaptic AMPA receptors using distinct SNARE-dependent mechanisms. Neuron. 2015;**86**(2):442-456

[19] Chen L, Lau AG, Sarti F. Synaptic retinoic acid signaling and homeostatic synaptic plasticity. Neuropharmacology. 2014;**78**:3-12

[20] Bonhomme D, Minni AM, Alfos S, Roux P, Richard E, Higueret P, et al. Vitamin A status regulates glucocorticoid availability in Wistar rats: Consequences on cognitive functions and hippocampal neurogenesis? Frontiers in Behavioral Neuroscience. 2014;**20**:1-13

[21] Bonnet E, Touyarot K, Alfos S, Pallet V, Higueret P, Abrous DN. Retinoic acid restores adult hippocampal neurogenesis and reverses spatial memory deficit in vitamin A deprived rats. In: McCabe BD, editor. PLoS One. 2008;**3**(10):e3487

[22] Jacobs S, Lie DC, DeCicco KL, Shi Y, DeLuca LM, Gage FH, et al. Retinoic acid is required early during adult neurogenesis in the dentate gyrus. Proceedings of the National Academy of Sciences of the United States of America. 2006;**103**(10):3902-3907

[23] Touyarot K, Bonhomme D, Roux P, Alfos S, Lafenêtre P, Richard E, et al. A mid-life vitamin A supplementation prevents age-related spatial memory deficits and hippocampal neurogenesis alterations through CRABP-I. PLoS One. 2013;**8**(8):e72101

[24] Hedden T, Gabrieli JDE. Insights into the ageing mind: A view from cognitive neuroscience. Nature Reviews. Neuroscience. 2004;**5**(2):87-96

[25] Bonhomme D, Pallet V, Dominguez G, Servant L, Henkous N, Lafenêtre P, et al. Retinoic acid modulates intrahippocampal levels of corticosterone in middle-aged mice: Consequences on hippocampal plasticity and contextual memory. Frontiers in Aging Neuroscience. 2014;**6**:6

[26] Etchamendy N, Enderlin V, Marighetto A, Pallet V, Higueret P, Jaffard R. Vitamin A deficiency and relational memory deficit in adult mice: Relationships with changes in brain retinoid signalling. Behavioural Brain Research. 2003;**145**(1-2):37-49

[27] Mingaud F, Mormede C, Etchamendy N, Mons N, Niedergang B, Wietrzych M, et al. Retinoid hyposignaling contributes to aging-related decline in hippocampal function in short-term/working memory organization and long-term declarative memory encoding in mice. Journal of Neuroscience: The Official Journal of the Society for Neuroscience. 2008;**28**(1):279-291

[28] Corcoran JPT, So PL, Maden M. Disruption of the retinoid signalling pathway causes a deposition of amyloid beta in the adult rat brain. The European Journal of Neuroscience. 2004;**20**(4):896-902

[29] Goncalves MB, Clarke E, Hobbs C, Malmqvist T, Deacon R, Jack J, et al. Amyloid β inhibits retinoic acid

synthesis exacerbating Alzheimer disease pathology which can be attenuated by an retinoic acid receptor α agonist. The European Journal of Neuroscience. 2013;**37**(7):1182-1192

[30] Goodman AB. Retinoid receptors, transporters, and metabolizers as therapeutic targets in late onset Alzheimer disease. Journal of Cellular Physiology. 2006;**209**(3):598-603

[31] Goodman AB, Pardee AB. Evidence for defective retinoid transport and function in late onset Alzheimer's disease. Proceedings of the National Academy of Sciences of the United States of America. 2003;**100**(5):2901-2905

[32] Sodhi RK, Singh N. Retinoids as potential targets for Alzheimer's disease. Pharmacology, Biochemistry, and Behavior. 2014;**120**:117-123

[33] Cai H, Liu G, Sun L, Ding J. Aldehyde dehydrogenase 1 making molecular inroads into the differential vulnerability of nigrostriatal dopaminergic neuron subtypes in Parkinson's disease. Translational Neurodegeneration. 2014;**3**:27

[34] Liu G, Yu J, Ding J, Xie C, Sun L, Rudenko I, et al. Aldehyde dehydrogenase 1 defines and protects a nigrostriatal dopaminergic neuron subpopulation. The Journal of Clinical Investigation. 2014;**124**(7):3032-3046

[35] Carta M, Stancampiano R, Tronci E, Collu M, Usiello A, Morelli M, et al. Vitamin A deficiency induces motor impairments and striatal cholinergic dysfunction in rats. Neuroscience. 2006;**139**(4):1163-1172

[36] Krezel W, Ghyselinck N, Samad TA, Dupé V, Kastner P, Borrelli E, et al. Impaired locomotion and dopamine signaling in retinoid receptor mutant mice. Science. 1998;**279**(5352):863-867

[37] Esteves M, Cristóvão AC, Saraiva T, Rocha SM, Baltazar G, Ferreira L, et al. Retinoic acid-loaded polymeric nanoparticles induce neuroprotection in a mouse model for Parkinson's disease. Frontiers in Aging Neuroscience. 2015;**7**:20

[38] Reiner DJ, Yu S-J, Shen H, He Y, Bae E, Wang Y. 9-cis retinoic acid protects against methamphetamine-induced neurotoxicity in nigrostriatal dopamine neurons. Neurotoxicity Research. 2014;**25**(3):248-261

Section 2

PUFA Metabolism in the Brain

Chapter 2

Polyunsaturated Fatty Acid Metabolism in the Brain and Brain Cells

Corinne Joffre

Abstract

Dietary polyunsaturated fatty acids (PUFAs) have gained more importance these last decades since they regulate the level of long-chain PUFAs (LC-PUFAs) in all cells and especially in brain cells. Because LC-PUFAs, especially those of the n-3 family, display both anti-inflammatory and pro-resolution properties, they play an essential role in neuroinflammation. Neuroinflammation is a hallmark of neurological disorders and requires to be tightly controlled or at least limited otherwise it can have functional consequences and negatively impact the quality of life and well-being of patients. LC-PUFAs exert these beneficial properties in part through the synthesis of specialized pro-resolving mediators (SPMs) that are involved in the resolution of inflammation and to the return of homeostasis. SPMs are promising relevant candidates to resolve brain inflammation and to contribute to neuroprotective functions and lead to novel therapeutics for brain inflammatory diseases. Here we present an overview of the origin and accumulation of PUFAs in the brain and brain cells and their conversion into SPMs that are involved in neuroinflammation and how nutrition induces variations in LC-PUFA and SPM levels in the brain and in brain cells.

Keywords: long-chain polyunsaturated fatty acids (LC-PUFAs), docosahexaenoic acid (DHA), eicosapentaenoic acid (EPA), specialized pro-resolving mediators (SPMs), nutrition, neuroinflammation, brain, brain cells

1. Introduction

Polyunsaturated fatty acids (PUFA) are essential fatty acids including precursors and long-chain PUFAs (LC-PUFAs). Precursors have to be provided by the diet because they cannot be produced by mammals [1]. They can be converted into LC-PUFAs. However, as the conversion rate is very low in human [2, 3], it is recommended to consume also LC-PUFAs that modulate LC-PUFA composition of brain and brain cells. Altered dietary intake and/or PUFA metabolism has been reported to be involved in a number of neurological disorders *via* sustained neuroinflammatory processes [4]. Indeed, LC-PUFAs are key regulators of inflammation [5]. LC-PUFAs can be metabolized into specific derivatives such as specialized pro-resolving mediators (SPMs) that have anti-inflammatory and pro-resolving properties [6–9], giving the LC-PUFAs and their biological derivatives a growing interest to treat inflammation and more specifically neuroinflammation. Hence, they may

 IntechOpen

represent a relevant alternative or complementary strategy to treat pathologies involving neuroinflammation. Here, we will review the literature on PUFAs and their bioactive lipid derivatives in the brain and brain cells. The book chapter will be divided in two main sections: in the first one, we will report data on the origin of PUFAs in the brain and on PUFA content in brain and brain cells and in the second one, we will review recent data on the bioactive lipid derivatives and their role in neuroinflammation. We will discuss how nutrition, an environmental factor to which individuals are exposed throughout their life, is a factor of variation of PUFA and their mediator contents in both sections. We will focus on total brain but also on brain cells since brain cells are differently affected by dietary supply.

2. PUFAs in the brain and brain cells

2.1 Origin of PUFAs in the brain

2.1.1 Metabolism of PUFAs

PUFAs are fatty acids containing more than one double bond on their carbon chain. They are classified into two main series, the n-6 PUFAs and the n-3 PUFAs depending on the position of the first double bond from the methyl terminal end. N-6 PUFAs have the first double bond at the 6th carbon and n-3 PUFAs at the 3rd. Of these two series, linoleic acid (LA) and alpha-linolenic acid (ALA) are the precursors and are essential fatty acids because mammals cannot synthesize them. *In vivo*, these precursors can be elongated, desaturated and beta-oxidized into fatty acids with additional double bonds and carbon atoms leading to long-chain PUFAs (LC-PUFAs, ≥20 carbon atoms) (**Figure 1**). This metabolic pathway requires specific Δ6 and Δ5 desaturases and elongases that are common to both n-6 and n-3 PUFAs, meaning that these pathways are in competition [10]. LC-PUFA

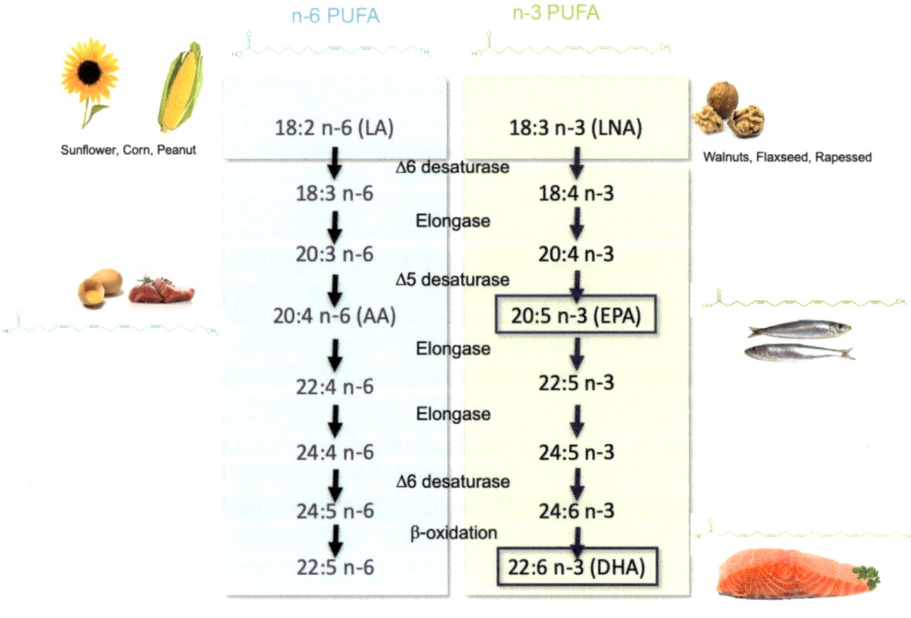

Figure 1.
Synthesis pathways of n-6 and n-3 LC-PUFA and main dietary sources of PUFAs. LA: linoleic acid; LNA: linolenic acid; AA: arachidonic acid; EPA: eicosapentaenoic acid; DHA: docosahexaenoic acid.

biosynthesis takes place mainly in the liver, especially in both microsomes and peroxisomes [11]. However, the brain also possesses the enzymatic equipment and can synthesize LC-PUFAs. The main LC-PUFAs for the n-6 and n-3 series, due to their role as precursors of bioactive derivatives and due to their level in the brain, are arachidonic acid (AA, 20:4 n-6) and docosahexaenoic acid (DHA, 22:6 n-3) [12, 13]. Eicosapentaenoic acid (EPA, 20:5 n-3) is also an important n-3 LC-PUFA as it is also a precursor of bioactive derivatives despite its low level in the brain because of its rapid β-oxidation [14]. Docosapentaenoic acid (DPA, 22:5 n-6) for the n-6 family is also relevant because it replaces DHA in the membranes in case of dietary n-3 PUFA deficiency. LC-PUFAs are mainly esterified in phospholipids. They are also present as free LC-PUFA in very low amount: 1 nmole/g tissue *versus* 10 μmoles/g [15].

2.1.2 Dietary origin

The precursors LA and ALA are found mainly in vegetables, oils, and seeds (60% of LA in sunflower oil and 10% of ALA in rapeseed oil, for example) (**Figure 1**) [16, 17]. Although human can synthesize LC-PUFAs from these precursors, the conversion efficiency is very low (<5%) even in healthy adults [2, 3]. Hence, the main part of LC-PUFAs comes from the diet. AA is found in meats (5–10%) and eggs (15%) [18, 19] and DHA and EPA are found in fatty fishes (18.7% EPA + DHA in salmon, 32.9% EPA + DHA in tuna, for example) (**Figure 1**) [20]. However, lean fishes (sole, codfish, etc.) contain also appreciable amounts of DHA and EPA. Therefore, LC-PUFAs dietary intakes are crucial to maintain adequate levels of LC-PUFAs in membranes. That is why there are dietary recommendations for PUFAs. Dietary intakes recommend ~500 mg/day in EPA and DHA (2 portions of fish/week) and a ratio LA/ALA close to 4–5 to meet all the needs of the body into DHA and to protect against cardiovascular disease risk [21, 22]. Preclinical and clinical studies indicate that increasing dietary ALA and reducing LA are beneficial in increasing n-3 LC-PUFA bioavailability [23, 24]. Despite these recommendations, dietary n-3 PUFA intake is insufficient, both for the precursor ALA and the LC-PUFAs DHA and EPA. Indeed, in the western diet, there is an imbalance between n-6 and n-3 PUFAs leading to an n-3 PUFA consumption 12–20 times lower than n-6 PUFA consumption [10, 25]. This is due to the increased industrialization in the developed nations accompanied by changes in dietary habits. It is particularly characterized by an increase in LA and AA together with a decrease in ALA and DHA. A high intake of LA associated with a low intake of ALA leads to the accumulation of n-6 PUFAs, including AA. In case of severe n-3 PUFA deficiency, the expression of desaturases and elongases are upregulated in the liver in order to compensate and provide DHA to the brain [26, 27]. In addition, under dietary n-3 PUFA deficiency, the half-life of brain DHA is increased by twofold as under balanced diet [28]. Dietary lipids, representing 35–40% of total energy intake, are essentially found (90–95%) in the form of triglycerides (a glycerol backbone with three fatty acids). They are also found in the form of phospholipids (in which the 3-position on the glycerol is replaced by a phosphorylated alcohol function). There is still a debate concerning the better form to enhance EPA/DHA bioavailability, krill oil as a source of phospholipids or fish oil as a source of triglycerides [29, 30]. More studies have to be performed.

2.2 PUFA content in the brain

The brain contains high levels of PUFAs (25–30%) that are mainly DHA (n-3 PUFA) (12–14% of total fatty acids) and AA (n-6 PUFA) (8–10% of total fatty acids) [12, 31–35]. Most LC-PUFAs accumulate during brain development, especially during the perinatal period: in humans between the beginning of the third trimester of gestation and 2 years and in rodents between the 7th and the 21st postnatal day [36–38]. These periods correspond to the rapid neuronal maturation, synaptogenesis, and gray matter expansion [39, 40]. The brain LC-PUFA content differs in brain structures [12, 31, 35, 41, 42], for example, in the adult C57Bl6/J mice, AA is higher in hippocampus (10.2%), followed by the prefrontal cortex (9.7%), the hypothalamus (8.5%), the cortex (7.7%), the cerebellum (6.5%), and the brain stem (5.5%) [12]. DHA is higher in the prefrontal cortex (14.3%) and in the hippocampus (13.7%), followed by cerebellum (12.2%) and cortex (11.9%), hypothalamus (10.1%), and brain stem (8.2%) [12]. Then the AA/DHA ratio varies from 0.75 to 0.85 in the hypothalamus and hippocampus to 0.54 in the cerebellum. These variations may be due to different LC-PUFA entry mechanisms into the brain or to different incorporation into membranes of cells composing the structure considered. These levels are comparable in human: prefrontal cortex contains between 12.3 and 15.9% of DHA in rats and mice and between 14.1 and 15.9% [12, 35, 43, 44].

2.3 PUFA content in brain cells

Brain cells comprise neurons and glial cells: 70% astrocytes, 10–15% oligodendrocytes, and 10–15% microglial cells [45]. Very few studies reported the fatty acid composition of the individual cells. Bourre et al. determined the fatty acid composition in neurons, astrocytes, and oligodendrocytes in 15- or 60-days rats and confirmed previous results obtained in 1973 and 1981 [46–49]. We recently described the fatty acid composition of microglial cells in 21-days mice [46, 50].

Neurons cannot synthesize LC-PUFAs but can incorporate them in their membranes. They contain 8.2–8.3% DHA and 2.2–2.8% n-3 DPA (22:5 n-3) for n-3 LC-PUFAs, 10.3–15.1% AA, 2.2% n-6 DPA, and 1.0–2.1% adrenic acid (22: 4 n-6) for n-6 LC-PUFAs [46]. They contain 3.1–6.9% LA. Then the ratio n-3/n-6 is 0.46–0.50.

Astrocytes are supportive glial cells that play many roles including synaptic transmission and energy metabolite furniture to different neural elements. They respond to all forms of central nervous system (CNS) insults through a process referred to as reactive astrogliosis. Dysfunctions of astrocytes result in pathological changes in the CNS. Astrocytes contain 10.6–12.1% DHA and 0.7–1.3% of n-3 DPA for n-3 LC-PUFAs and 10.1–10.3% of AA, 2.5–2.7% of n-6 DPA and 2.4–2.7% adrenic acid (22:4 n-6) [46]. They contain few PUFA precursors: only 1.2–1.4% of LA and no ALA. The ratio n-3/n-6 is 0.72–0.76.

Oligodendrocytes provide a supporting role for neurons and are involved in the formation of myelin sheaths of nerve cell axons. They are highly dynamic and can respond to environmental influences and neuronal activity. They can also regenerate myelin spontaneously after CNS injury. Any disturbances in their functioning are associated with major diseases of the nervous system. They contain mainly 5.1% DHA for n-3 LC-PUFAs and 9.3% AA and 3.5% n-6 DPA for n-6 LC-PUFAs [46]. They contain not as much as LA: only 2.7%. The ratio n-3/n-6 is 0.33.

Microglial cells are the innate immune cells of the brain. They play a major role in synaptogenesis, synapse structure and function, and neuroinflammation. They perpetually scan and control their environment and once activated, they deliver pro-inflammatory and pro-regeneration responses. Their fatty acid composition differs from that of the other brain cells. In all these cells, DHA is the main fatty acid. Microglial cells are characterized by few DHA (<1%) and n-3 DPA (0.1%) but high content of EPA (3.7%) [50]. They contain few AA (1.6%). They contain PUFA precursors: 8.0% LA and 1.3% ALA. The ratio n-3/n-6 is 0.42. This microglial fatty acid composition also differs from the whole brain hippocampus that contains higher DHA than EPA [51]. Then, it seems that EPA metabolism is different in microglial cells than in other brain cells and the whole brain structure. It is not highly β-oxidized as in the whole brain [52]. More studies have to be performed to elucidate the role of EPA in microglial cells.

2.4 Nutrition as a major factor of variation of brain and brain cell PUFA content

Nutrition is an environmental factor to which individuals are continuously exposed throughout life. And it is an environmental factor that changed a lot these last decades. Indeed, there was a dramatic reduction in the dietary supply of n-3 PUFAs in western societies associated with a drastic increase in the n-6 PUFAs, leading to an imbalanced n-6/n-3 PUFA ratio estimated at 12–20 in developed countries instead of five recommended [10].

This is particularly important considering that brain fatty acid composition varies with the fatty acids of the dietary supply [53]. Indeed, PUFA content is strongly impacted by the dietary PUFAs in all brain structures [12, 54]. A diet deficient in n-3 PUFA precursor during development and/or adulthood decreases brain DHA in all brain structures; the prefrontal cortex and the hippocampus that contain the highest DHA content are the most sensitive whereas the hypothalamus that contains the lowest DHA, is the least sensitive [12, 31, 55–58]. These differences may be attributed to the evolution of brain performance [59, 60]. In such case of n-3 PUFA deficiency, changes in metabolism occur: the half-life of DHA increases in the brain to reduce its loss [61] and the activity of DHA synthesis enzymes (Δ6 destaurase and elongase) is increased in the liver [26, 62, 63]. In contrast to the deficiency, the supplementation in n-3 LC-PUFAs increases brain DHA [64–67]. DHA supplementation is more efficient than ALA supplementation to increase brain DHA [68, 69]. A DHA supplementation is also efficient to reverse brain DHA decrease due to an n-3 PUFA deficiency or to aging [33, 70–72]. Also, genetic models of n-3 PUFA enrichment such as Fat-1 mice possess higher brain DHA content [12, 73–77].

Brain cells are also impacted by dietary PUFA supply. An n-3 PUFA precursor-deficient diet decreases DHA in neurons (4.6% *versus* 8.2% in 15-day old animals and 2.4 *versus* 8.3% in 60-day old animals), astrocytes (3.1 *versus* 10.6% in 15-day old animals and 5.7 *versus* 12.1% in 60-day old animals), and oligodendrocytes (0.1% *versus* 5.1% in 60-day old animals) [46]. These changes decrease the n-3/n-6 ratio (0.24 *versus* 0.46–0.50 in neurons, 0.12–0.25 *versus* 0.72–0.76 in astrocytes and 0.02 *versus* 0.33 in oligodendrocytes). Interestingly, we recently find that a maternal n-3 PUFA precursor deficiency increases n-6 DPA but does not affect DHA level in microglial cells in 21-day-old animals, suggesting that these cells are protected from n-3 PUFA deficiency [50]. However, we also report that a maternal n-3 LC-PUFA supplementation increases DHA levels and decreases n-6 DPA levels in these animals, confirming results previously obtained in glial cells [78, 79].

All these results suggest that brain DHA levels are highly variables, depending on the brain structures or brain cells considered and on the dietary fatty acid intake. This may have consequences on inflammatory processes since n-3 LC-PUFAs have immunomodulatory properties [80].

3. Bioactive PUFA derivatives

3.1 Bioactive PUFA derivative metabolism

3.1.1 PUFA derivative synthesis pathways

Some of the immunomodulatory properties of LC-PUFAs are attributed to the synthesis of bioactive lipid mediators. Different lipid mediators are synthesized: those involved in the regulation of inflammation such as the eicosanoids (prostaglandins, leukotrienes, and thromboxanes) and those implicated in the resolution of inflammation called specialized pro-resolving mediators (SPMs, resolvins, protectins, and maresins) (**Figure 2**). Among the eicosanoids, those synthesized from n-3 PUFAs are less potent inflammatory than those synthesized from n-6 PUFAs [81] highlighting the interest to increase n-3 PUFA and decrease n-6 PUFA contents in the membranes. Then, when co-present, EPA-derived eicosanoids antagonize those synthesized from AA. The main EPA-derived mediators include 3-series prostaglandin (PG), 5-series leukotriene (LT), and 3-series thromboxane (TX), reported to be nonactive (**Figure 2**). DHA is also converted into 3-series PG (**Figure 2**). In addition, eicosanoids synthesized from AA and EPA act in competition as they share the same G-protein-coupled receptors. Moreover, EPA is a competitive inhibitor to AA. Indeed, it reduces the production of AA by inhibiting the activity of Δ5 desaturase converting dihomo-gamma-linolenic acid (dGLA) into AA [81]. EPA also reduces *in vitro* the production of AA-derived eicosanoids by inhibiting the activity of cyclooxygenase-2 (COX-2) and 5-lipoxygenase (5-LOX) generating the eicosanoids [82–84]. Eicosanoids are synthesized first in the time course of the inflammatory response. Then, there is a switch in the bioactive lipid mediator class: SPMs derived from n-3 LC-PUFAs are synthesized to induce the resolution of inflammation and a return to homeostasis (**Figure 3**). DHA is the precursor of D-series resolvins, neuroprotectin D1 (NPD1), and Maresin 1–2 (Mar1–2) and EPA is the precursor of E-series resolvins, all these derivatives underlying most of the beneficial effects attributed to their precursors [1, 85–87]. These derivatives have both anti-inflammatory and pro-resolution properties without immune suppression [6, 8, 88, 89]. SPMs actively orchestrate and finely tune the inflammatory response. They decrease pro-inflammatory cytokines and increase anti-inflammatory cytokines and accelerate the phagocytosis of cellular debris and dead cells without immune suppression. They are synthesized *via* COX-2, LOX, and cytochrome P450 monooxygenases (CYP450) once they have been released from membrane phospholipids by phospholipase A2 in response to stimulation. These

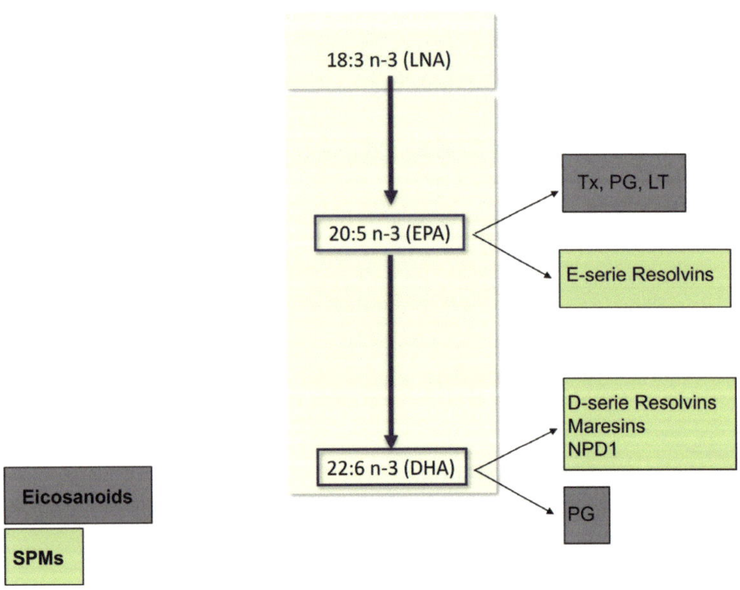

Figure 2.
Main bioactive lipid mediators synthesized from n-3 PUFAs. DHA: docosahexaenoic acid; EPA: eicosapentaenoic acid; LNA: linolenic acid; LT: leukotriene; NPD1: neuroprotection D1; PG: prostaglandin; SPMs: specialized pro-resolving mediators; Tx: thromboxane.

enzymes are expressed in the brain [90–92]. In response to lipopolysaccharide (LPS) that induces inflammation, COX-2 is rapidly expressed in the hippocampus [69, 93] and inhibition of COX-2 delays resolution of acute inflammation [94]. 15-LOX and 5-LOX are the most abundant LOX in the brain [90]. 15-LOX has a dual role since it is involved in neurodegeneration and neurotoxicity due to the increased stress it generates [95–97] and is also involved in neuroprotection [98]. 15-LOX deletion or inhibition decreases SPM production in the brain and cognitive alterations [90]. CYP450 generates n-6 derived epoxides that are anti-inflammatory [99–102]. These enzymes are also expressed in microglia, astrocytes, oligodendrocytes, and neurons [103–106].

3.1.2 Bioactive lipid mediators

DHA is converted into monohydroxy DHA (17-HDHA) by acetylated COX-2, CYP450, and 15-LOX [107, 108] and then into RvD1 by 5-LOX [109, 110]. RvD1 and its precursors have mostly been described at the periphery but have also been detected in the brain. RvD1 was measured in mouse brain following cerebral ischemia. Its level is increased following a DHA intravenous injection [111] and modulated during inflammation: it decreases at the beginning and then increases during the resolution phase [112]. RvD1 acts through the regulation of micro-RNAs (miRNAs) that modulate the expression of target genes such as inflammatory genes [113–117]. DHA can also be converted into di-hydroxy-DHA termed protectin D1 (PD1) or neuroprotectin D1 (NPD1) when produced in the CNS by 5- and 15-LOX [118–121]. NPD1 was measured in hippocampus. Its level greatly is increased following brain ischemia or acute central LPS injection [70, 122] and decreased in the hippocampus of Alzheimer's disease patients [123]. NPD1 acts through NFkB and then decreases pro-inflammatory gene expression [122, 124, 125]. At last, DHA can also be converted into 14-HDHA and then in Mar1–2 by 12/15-LOX [107, 108, 126]. Mar1 and its precursor 14-HDHA have recently been identified in the hippocampus of mice [70]. Its level is decreased in post-mortem Alzheimer's disease patients contributing to the progression of this pathology [127]. Mar1 promotes the resolution of inflammation, reducing pro-inflammatory cytokines, silencing pro-inflammatory signaling cascades, and enhancing M2 repair macrophage phenotype after cerebral ischemia or spinal cord injury [128–130] (**Figure 3**).

EPA is converted into resolvins E1, E2, and E3 by acetylated COX-2 or CYP450 *via* 18R-HEPE by 5- or 15-LOX [107, 131, 132]. RvE1 and its precursor have been detected in hippocampus [70, 133, 134]. RvE1 inhibits NFκB signaling pathway and then decreases LPS-induced proinflammatory cytokines (TNF-α, IL-6, and IL-1β) gene expression in microglial cells [117].

3.1.3 SPM receptors

SPMs act through specific receptors, some but not all of them have recently been identified. RvD1 acts through lipoxin A4 receptor/formyl peptide receptor 2 (ALX/Fpr2) in rodents and G protein coupling receptor 32 (GPR32) in human [109] at picomolar range but induces biological effects at nanomolar range [110, 135]. RvE1 directly binds to its receptor G protein coupling receptor ChemR23 or chemokine like receptor 1 (CMKLR1) [131]. It is also a partial agonist of a leukotriene B4 receptor (BLT1) [136]. In the CNS, ALX/Fpr2 has been identified in the brainstem, spinal cord, hypothalamus, cortex, hippocampus, cerebellum, and striatum [137] and ChemR23 in the prefrontal cortex, hippocampus, and brainstem [138]. At the cellular levels, these two receptors have been detected in microglial cells [117, 139], neurons [137, 140] and astrocytes [96, 113] (**Figure 3**).

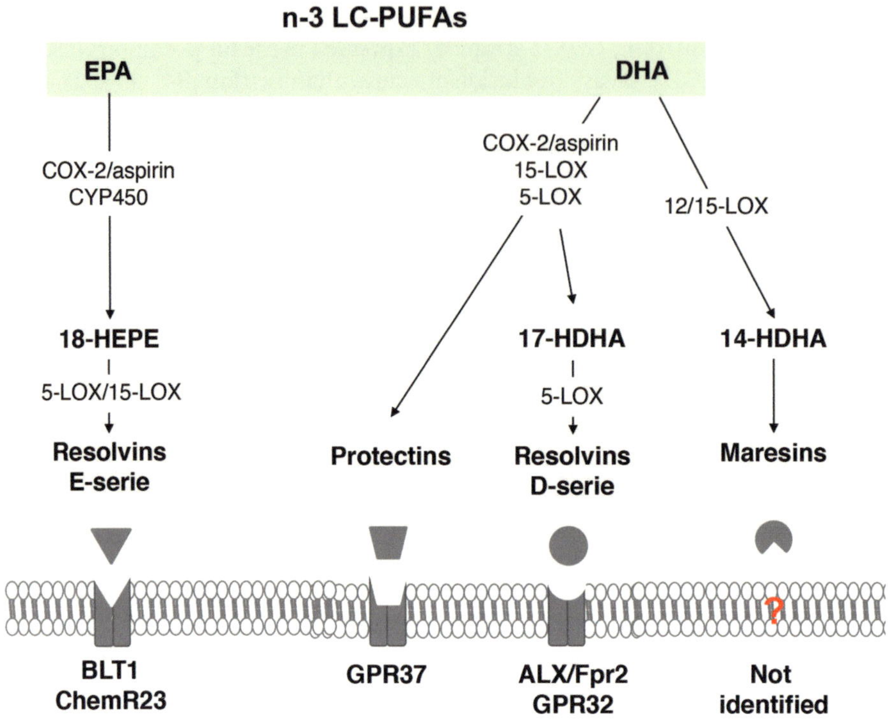

Figure 3.
Specialized pro-resolving mediator (SPM) synthesis. 14-HDHA: 14-hydroxy-docosahexaenoic acid; 17-HDHA: 17-hydroxy-docosahexaenoic acid; 18-HEPE: 18-hydroxy-eicosapentaenoic acid; ALX/Fpr2: N-formyl peptide receptor 2; BLT1: leukotriene B4 receptor; COX-2: cyclooxygenases; DHA: docosahexaenoic acid; EPA: eicosapentaenoic acid; GPR32/37: G protein-coupled receptor 32/37; LC-PUFAs: long chain polyunsaturated fatty acids; LOX: lipoxygenases.

Other receptors have not been identified yet (Mar1 receptor) [127] or identified only at the periphery in macrophages but not in microglia (NPD1 receptor) [141].

In the next sections, we will focus on the role of these SPMs to better understand the beneficial effects of the n-3 PUFAs.

3.2 Role of bioactive lipid derivatives in neuroinflammation

SPMs have multiple biological roles, focusing to the return to homeostasis. In human serum, DHA- and EPA-derivatives represent 30.7 and 25.9% of the identified SPMs, respectively [142, 143]. The most SPMs studied are RvD1 and RvE1 because they have powerful anti-inflammatory and pro-resolution properties. We will then detail the biological roles for these two bioactive mediators.

3.2.1 Biological role of RvD1 and RvE1 in humans

The effect of RvD1 was mainly studied in patients suffering from Alzheimer's disease. Interestingly, RvD1 levels in cerebrospinal fluid are positively correlated with the enhancement of cognitive functions of patients with dementia [96]. Moreover, it was suggested *in vitro* in macrophages isolated from Alzheimer's patients that RvD1 may be involved in Aβ phagocytosis [144, 145]. Then the decrease in RvD1 levels in Alzheimer's patient brain could contribute to the disease development. To our knowledge, the effect of RvE1 in humans was shown at the periphery (on patients undergoing hepatobiliary resection, pulmonary inflammation, and bone disease periodontitis) [146–148] but not at the brain level on patients suffering from neurodegenerative diseases.

3.2.2 Biological roles of RvD1 and RvE1 in rodents

RvD1 and RvE1 are active in reducing the pro-inflammatory status in the CNS. Indeed, the precursors of RvD1, 17R-HDHA, and 17S-HDHA decrease the production of pro-inflammatory cytokines TNF-α in the spinal cord and IL-1β and TNF-α in the hippocampus [70, 149]. Moreover, RvD1 is able to induce the polarization of macrophages and microglia toward an M2 phagocytic phenotype [150–152]. In addition, RvD1 reduces neuroinflammation *via* miRNA in a model of remote damage [113]. RvE1 also modulates inflammation by reducing the proinflammatory cytokines IL-1β and IL-6 in the prefrontal cortex and decreases the measures of Aβ pathology in a murine model of Alzheimer's disease [153]. Furthermore, RvE1 treatment decreases brain microglial activation following traumatic brain injury or peripheral brain injury, decreasing the proportion of activated microglia at the expense of ramified microglia [154, 155].

RvD1 is also involved in the prevention of cognitive deficits. In a systemic inflammation model, cognitive decline is prevented by an intraperitoneal (ip) injection of the precursor of RvD1, 17R-HDHA, and is associated with the restoration of transmission and synaptic plasticity and to the prevention of astrogliosis [154, 156]. Moreover, in a model of traumatic brain injury, cognitive deficits are also prevented by an ip chronic administration of 17R-HDHA [154]. Of note, Fat-1 mice that have more brain n-3 LC-PUFAs have higher hippocampus RvD1 that is associated with less cognitive deficits, a better neuronal survival, a decrease in astrocyte and microglial activation and a reduction in pro-inflammatory status following brain ischemia [77, 157]. Inversely, an inhibition of 15-LOX associated with a decrease in RvD1 induces alterations in synaptic plasticity and working memory [90].

Additionally, RvD and E are also associated with the prevention of depressive-like behaviors [158]. An intracerebroventricular (icv) injection of RvD1, D2, E1, E2, or E3 significantly decreases LPS-induced depressive-like behaviors [159–161]. Moreover, an intrathecal injection of 17R-HDHA prevents the occurrence of depressive-like behaviors and is associated with the decrease of pain perception and a restoration of dopamine and glutamate levels in the brain [149, 162]. RvD1 and D2 have also positive effects in chronic mild stress-induced depression and in post-myocardial infarct depression [163, 164].

3.2.3 Biological roles of RvD1 and RvE1 in in vitro brain cell models

The effects of RvD1 were tested on different brain cells. In microglial cells, RvD1 potentiates the activation of the anti-inflammatory M2 phenotype of microglia, enhancing the effect of the anti-inflammatory cytokine IL-4, Arg1, and Ym1 expression and decreasing CD11b expression [152, 155, 165]. Moreover, we showed that RvD1 decreases LPS-induced proinflammatory cytokine (TNF-α, IL-6 and IL-1β) gene expression in microglial BV2 cells *via* the modulation of miRNAs [117]. RvD2 inhibits LPS-induced activation of toll-like receptor 4 (TLR4, the receptor of LPS) and its downstream signaling pathway NFκB [166]. RvE1 plays also a direct role in microglial cells by inhibiting microglial activation and pro-inflammatory cytokine release [117, 155]. These results suggest the pro-resolution activity of RvD1 and RvE1 in microglia. In astrocytes, RvD1 decreases TNF-α release induced by LPS injection [149]. In neurons from spinal nods, RvD1 increases neurite outgrowth [167].

All these studies point out the central role of n-3 LC-PUFA and their bioactive mediators in the regulation of inflammation in the brain, especially through their effect on microglia.

3.3 Nutrition as a factor of variation of SPM levels

The level of these lipid derivatives is modulated by the diet. Indeed, we recently show that a dietary n-3 LC-PUFA supplementation induces an n-3 LC-PUFA enrichment in the hippocampus associated with an increase in n-3 PUFA-derived SPMs and a decrease in n-6 PUFA-derived SPMs [69]. Our results confirm previous ones reporting that oral administration of EPA and DHA results in the generation of EPA-and DHA-derived mediators in the cortex of aged rats [168] and in the down-regulation of the production of n-6 PUFA-derived mediators [169, 170]. The cellular origin of these bioactive lipid derivatives is still unknown. As described in the paragraph above, we know that dietary PUFA supplementation affects PUFA composition in brain cells that potentially could impact brain cell PUFA lipid derivatives. In response to LPS, n-3 LC-PUFA-supplemented mice display an anti-inflammatory SPM profile whereas n-3 LC-PUFA-deficient mice exhibit a pro-inflammatory SPM profile [69]. These results corroborate previous ones *in vivo* [171–176] and *in vitro* in macrophages [177, 178] and microglia [179–181].

The level of SPMs is also dependent on the regulation of their biosynthesis enzymes. 15-LOX mRNA expression increases in n-3 LC-PUFA supplemented group and decreases in n-3 LC-PUFA deficient diet [27, 69, 182]. 15-LOX has beneficial properties such as neuroprotective properties *via* PPAR-γ activation [98] and preservation of cognitive performance through RvD1 formation [90]. 15-LOX has also detrimental effects as it is implicated in neurodegeneration and neurotoxicity through increase of oxidative stress [95–97].

Changes in SPM level and composition induced by the diet can have a great influence on the pro- and anti-inflammatory status of hippocampus and brain cells and reinforce the recommendation of n-3 PUFA-rich diet.

4. Conclusion

These data highlight that n-3 LC-PUFA and their bioactive lipid derivatives are important regulators of neuroinflammation. SPMs are promising therapeutic compounds: they are of natural origin and act in physiologic dose ranges (nanomolar) as compared to EPA and DHA that act at micromolar ranges, and this confers the main advantage to use SPMs. Both brain n-3 LC-PUFA and SPMs are modulated by the diet in the brain and in brain cells confirming the notable role of nutrition in the regulation of inflammation. Alteration in dietary n-3 PUFAs should have dramatic consequences in brain and brain cell PUFA metabolism and finally in the response to neuroinflammation. The use of SPMs to treat neuroinflammation is still in emergence since some data are missing such as the affinity and function of SPM receptors. This field has to be completed. The instability of SPMs may be bypassed by the use of SPM analogues or by their encapsulation. The clinical form and the way of administration should also be defined.

Acknowledgements

Corinne Joffre was sponsored by the Fondation de France and the Fondation pour la Recherche Médicale.

Author details

Corinne Joffre[1,2]

1 INRA, Nutrition et Neurobiologie Intégrée, UMR 1286, Bordeaux, France

2 Université de Bordeaux 2, Bordeaux Cedex, France

*Address all correspondence to: corinne.joffre@inra.fr

References

[1] Bazinet RP, Layé S. Polyunsaturated fatty acids and their metabolites in brain function and disease. Nature Reviews. Neuroscience. Dec. 2014;**15**(12):771-785

[2] Kidd PM. Omega-3 DHA and EPA for cognition, behavior, and mood: Clinical findings and structural-functional synergies with cell membrane phospholipids. Alternative Medicine Review. Sep. 2007;**12**(3):207-227

[3] Plourde M, Cunnane SC. Extremely limited synthesis of long chain polyunsaturates in adults: Implications for their dietary essentiality and use as supplements. Applied Physiology, Nutrition, and Metabolism. Aug. 2007;**32**(4):619-634

[4] Dantzer R, O'Connor JC, Freund GG, Johnson RW, Kelley KW. From inflammation to sickness and depression: When the immune system subjugates the brain. Nature Reviews. Neuroscience. Jan. 2008;**9**(1):46-56

[5] Calder PC. Marine omega-3 fatty acids and inflammatory processes: Effects, mechanisms and clinical relevance. Biochimica et Biophysica Acta. Apr. 2015;**1851**(4):469-484

[6] Serhan CN, Clish CB, Brannon J, Colgan SP, Chiang N, Gronert K. Novel functional sets of lipid-derived mediators with antiinflammatory actions generated from omega-3 fatty acids via cyclooxygenase 2-nonsteroidal antiinflammatory drugs and transcellular processing. The Journal of Experimental Medicine. Oct. 2000;**192**(8):1197-1204

[7] Serhan CN. The resolution of inflammation: The devil in the flask and in the details. The FASEB Journal. May 2011;**25**(5):1441-1448

[8] Serhan CN. Pro-resolving lipid mediators are leads for resolution physiology. Nature. Jun. 2014;**510**(7503):92-101

[9] Spite M, Serhan CN. Novel lipid mediators promote resolution of acute inflammation: Impact of aspirin and statins. Circulation Research. Nov. 2010;**107**(10):1170-1184

[10] Simopoulos AP. Evolutionary aspects of diet: The omega-6/omega-3 ratio and the brain. Molecular Neurobiology. Oct. 2011;**44**(2):203-215

[11] Sprecher H. Metabolism of highly unsaturated n-3 and n-6 fatty acids. Biochimica et Biophysica Acta. Jul. 2000;**1486**(2-3):219-231

[12] Joffre C et al. Modulation of brain PUFA content in different experimental models of mice. Prostaglandins, Leukotrienes, and Essential Fatty Acids. 2016;**114**:1-10

[13] Kitajka K et al. Effects of dietary omega-3 polyunsaturated fatty acids on brain gene expression. Proceedings of the National Academy of Sciences of the United States of America. Jul. 2004;**101**(30):10931-10936

[14] Chen CT, Bazinet RP. beta-oxidation and rapid metabolism, but not uptake regulate brain eicosapentaenoic acid levels. Prostaglandins, Leukotrienes, and Essential Fatty Acids. Jan. 2015;**92**:33-40

[15] Green JT, Liu Z, Bazinet RP. Brain phospholipid arachidonic acid half-lives are not altered following 15 weeks of N-3 polyunsaturated fatty acid adequate or deprived diet. Journal of Lipid Research. Mar. 2010;**51**(3):535-543

[16] Orsavova J, Misurcova L, Ambrozova JV, Vicha R, Mlcek J. Fatty acids composition of vegetable oils and its contribution to dietary energy intake and dependence of cardiovascular

mortality on dietary intake of fatty acids. International Journal of Molecular Sciences. Jun. 2015;**16**(6):12871-12890

[17] Lewinska A, Zebrowski J, Duda M, Gorka A, Wnuk M. Fatty acid profile and biological activities of linseed and rapeseed oils. Molecules. Dec. 2015;**20**(12):22872-22880

[18] Meyer BJ, Mann NJ, Lewis JL, Milligan GC, Sinclair AJ, Howe PRC. Dietary intakes and food sources of omega-6 and omega-3 polyunsaturated fatty acids. Lipids. Apr. 2003;**38**(4):391-398

[19] Taber L, Chiu CH, Whelan J. Assessment of the arachidonic acid content in foods commonly consumed in the American diet. Lipids. Dec. 1998;**33**(12):1151-1157

[20] Strobel C, Jahreis G, Kuhnt K. Survey of n-3 and n-6 polyunsaturated fatty acids in fish and fish products. Lipids in Health and Disease. Oct. 2012;**11**:144

[21] Burdge G. Alpha-linolenic acid metabolism in men and women: Nutritional and biological implications. Current Opinion in Clinical Nutrition and Metabolic Care. Mar. 2004;**7**(2):137-144

[22] Lucas M, Asselin G, Mérette C, Poulin M-J, Dodin S. Validation of an FFQ for evaluation of EPA and DHA intake. Public Health Nutrition. Oct. 2009;**12**(10):1783-1790

[23] Blanchard H, Pédrono F, Boulier-Monthéan N, Catheline D, Rioux V, Legrand P. Comparative effects of well-balanced diets enriched in α-linolenic or linoleic acids on LC-PUFA metabolism in rat tissues. Prostaglandins, Leukotrienes, and Essential Fatty Acids. May 2013;**88**(5):383-389

[24] Taha AY et al. Dietary omega-6 fatty acid lowering increases bioavailability of omega-3 polyunsaturated fatty acids in human plasma lipid pools. Prostaglandins, Leukotrienes, and Essential Fatty Acids. May 2014;**90**(5):151-157

[25] Simopoulos AP. The importance of the ratio of omega-6/omega-3 essential fatty acids. Biomedicine & Pharmacotherapy. Oct. 2002;**56**(8):365-379

[26] Igarashi M, Ma K, Chang L, Bell JM, Rapoport SI. Dietary n-3 PUFA deprivation for 15 weeks upregulates elongase and desaturase expression in rat liver but not brain. Journal of Lipid Research. Nov. 2007;**48**(11):2463-2470

[27] Rao JS, Ertley RN, DeMar JC, Rapoport SI, Bazinet RP, Lee H-J. Dietary n-3 PUFA deprivation alters expression of enzymes of the arachidonic and docosahexaenoic acid cascades in rat frontal cortex. Molecular Psychiatry. Feb. 2007;**12**(2):151-157

[28] DeMar JC Jr, Ma K, Bell JM, Rapoport SI. Half-lives of docosahexaenoic acid in rat brain phospholipids are prolonged by 15 weeks of nutritional deprivation of n-3 polyunsaturated fatty acids. Journal of Neurochemistry. Dec. 2004;**91**(5):1125-1137

[29] Salem N, Kuratko CN. A reexamination of krill oil bioavailability studies. Lipids in Health and Disease. Aug. 2014;**13**:137

[30] Yurko-Mauro K, Kralovec J, Bailey-Hall E, Smeberg V, Stark JG, Salem N. Similar eicosapentaenoic acid and docosahexaenoic acid plasma levels achieved with fish oil or krill oil in a randomized double-blind four-week bioavailability study. Lipids in Health and Disease. Sep. 2015;**14**:99

[31] Carrie I, Clement M, de Javel D, Frances H, Bourre JM. Specific phospholipid fatty acid composition

of brain regions in mice. Effects of n-3 polyunsaturated fatty acid deficiency and phospholipid supplementation. Journal of Lipid Research. Mar. 2000;**41**(3):465-472

[32] Chung WL, Chen JJ, Su HM. Fish oil supplementation of control and (n-3) fatty acid-deficient male rats enhances reference and working memory performance and increases brain regional docosahexaenoic acid levels. The Journal of Nutrition. Jun. 2008;**138**(6):1165-1171

[33] Little SJ, Lynch MA, Manku M, Nicolaou A. Docosahexaenoic acid-induced changes in phospholipids in cortex of young and aged rats: A lipidomic analysis. Prostaglandins, Leukotrienes, and Essential Fatty Acids. Oct. 2007;**77**(3-4):155-162

[34] McNamara RK, Carlson SE. Role of omega-3 fatty acids in brain development and function: Potential implications for the pathogenesis and prevention of psychopathology. Prostaglandins, Leukotrienes, and Essential Fatty Acids. Oct. 2006;**75**(4-5):329-349

[35] Xiao Y, Huang Y, Chen ZY. Distribution, depletion and recovery of docosahexaenoic acid are region-specific in rat brain. The British Journal of Nutrition. Oct. 2005;**94**(4):544-550

[36] Clandinin MT, Chappell JE, Leong S, Heim T, Swyer PR, Chance GW. Extrauterine fatty acid accretion in infant brain: Implications for fatty acid requirements. Early Human Development. Jun. 1980;**4**(2):131-138

[37] Clandinin MT, Chappell JE, Leong S, Heim T, Swyer PR, Chance GW. Intrauterine fatty acid accretion rates in human brain: Implications for fatty acid requirements. Early Human Development. Jun. 1980;**4**(2):121-129

[38] Green P, Glozman S, Kamensky B, Yavin E. Developmental changes in rat brain membrane lipids and fatty acids. The preferential prenatal accumulation of docosahexaenoic acid. Journal of Lipid Research. May 1999;**40**(5):960-966

[39] Giedd JN et al. Brain development during childhood and adolescence: A longitudinal MRI study. Nature Neuroscience. Oct. 1999;**2**(10):861-863

[40] Morgane PJ et al. Prenatal malnutrition and development of the brain. Neuroscience and Biobehavioral Reviews. Spring 1993;**17**(1):91-128

[41] Delion S, Chalon S, Hérault J, Guilloteau D, Besnard JC, Durand G. Chronic dietary alpha-linolenic acid deficiency alters dopaminergic and serotoninergic neurotransmission in rats. The Journal of Nutrition. Dec. 1994;**124**(12):2466-2476

[42] McNamara RK, Able J, Jandacek R, Rider T, Tso P. Inbred C57BL/6J and DBA/2J mouse strains exhibit constitutive differences in regional brain fatty acid composition. Lipids. Jan. 2009;**44**(1):1-8

[43] Moriguchi T, Loewke J, Garrison M, Catalan JN, Salem N Jr. Reversal of docosahexaenoic acid deficiency in the rat brain, retina, liver, and serum. Journal of Lipid Research. Mar. 2001;**42**(3):419-427

[44] Hamazaki K, Maekawa M, Toyota T, Dean B, Hamazaki T, Yoshikawa T. Fatty acid composition of the postmortem prefrontal cortex of patients with schizophrenia, bipolar disorder, and major depressive disorder. Psychiatry Research. Jun. 2015;**227**(2-3):353-359

[45] Renaud J, Therien HM, Plouffe M, Martinoli MG. Neuroinflammation: Dr Jekyll or Mr Hyde? Medical Science (Paris). Nov. 2015;**31**(11):979-988

[46] Bourre JM, Pascal G, Durand G, Masson M, Dumont O, Piciotti M. Alterations in the fatty acid composition of rat brain cells (neurons, astrocytes, and oligodendrocytes) and of subcellular fractions (myelin and synaptosomes) induced by a diet devoid of n-3 fatty acids. Journal of Neurochemistry. Aug. 1984;**43**(2):342-348

[47] Cohen SR, Bernsohn J. Incorporation of 1-^{14}C labeled fatty acids into isolated neuronal soma, astroglia and oligodendroglia from calf brain. Brain Research;**60**(2):521-525

[48] Morand O, Masson M, Baumann N, Bourre JM. Exogenous [1-^{14}C]lignoceric acid uptake by neurons, astrocytes and myelin, as compared to incorporation of [1-^{14}C]palmitic and stearic acids. Neurochemistry International. 1981;**3**(5):329-334

[49] Morand O et al. Alteration in fatty acid composition of neurons, astrocytes, oligodendrocytes, myelin and synaptosomes in intrauterine malnutrition in rat. Annals of Nutrition & Metabolism. 1982;**26**(2):111-120

[50] Rey C et al. Maternal n-3 polyunsaturated fatty acid dietary supply modulates microglia lipid content in the offspring. Prostaglandins, Leukotrienes, and Essential Fatty Acids. 2018;**133**:1-7

[51] Madore C et al. Nutritional n-3 PUFAs deficiency during perinatal periods alters brain innate immune system and neuronal plasticity-associated genes. Brain, Behavior, and Immunity. Oct. 2014;**41**:22-31

[52] Chen CT, Liu Z, Ouellet M, Calon F, Bazinet RP. Rapid beta-oxidation of eicosapentaenoic acid in mouse brain: An in situ study. Prostaglandins, Leukotrienes, and Essential Fatty Acids. Feb. 2009;**80**(2-3):157-163

[53] Calder PC. Immunomodulation by omega-3 fatty acids. Prostaglandins, Leukotrienes, and Essential Fatty Acids. Dec. 2007;**77**(5-6):327-335

[54] Alashmali SM, Hopperton KE, Bazinet RP. Lowering dietary n-6 polyunsaturated fatty acids: Interaction with brain arachidonic and docosahexaenoic acids. Current Opinion in Lipidology. Feb. 2016;**27**(1):54-66

[55] Connor WE, Neuringer M, Lin DS. Dietary effects on brain fatty acid composition: The reversibility of n-3 fatty acid deficiency and turnover of docosahexaenoic acid in the brain, erythrocytes, and plasma of rhesus monkeys. Journal of Lipid Research. Feb. 1990;**31**(2):237-247

[56] Larrieu T, Madore C, Joffre C, Layé S. Nutritional n-3 polyunsaturated fatty acids deficiency alters cannabinoid receptor signaling pathway in the brain and associated anxiety-like behavior in mice. Journal of Physiology and Biochemistry. Dec. 2012;**68**(4):671-681

[57] Delpech J-C et al. Dietary n-3 PUFAs deficiency increases vulnerability to inflammation-induced spatial memory impairment. Neuropsychopharmacology. Nov. 2015;**40**(12):2774-2787

[58] Manduca A et al. Amplification of mGlu5-endocannabinoid signaling rescues behavioral and synaptic deficits in a mouse model of adolescent and adult dietary polyunsaturated fatty acid imbalance. Journal of Neuroscience;**37**(29):6851-6868

[59] Broadhurst CL, Wang Y, Crawford MA, Cunnane SC, Parkington JE, Schmidt WF. Brain-specific lipids from marine, lacustrine, or terrestrial food resources: Potential impact on early African *Homo sapiens*. Comparative Biochemistry and Physiology. Part B, Biochemistry & Molecular Biology. Apr. 2002;**131**(4):653-673

[60] Crawford MA et al. Evidence for the unique function of docosahexaenoic acid during the evolution of the modern hominid brain. Lipids. 1999;**34**(Suppl):S39-S47

[61] Rapoport SI, Rao JS, Igarashi M. Brain metabolism of nutritionally essential polyunsaturated fatty acids depends on both the diet and the liver. Prostaglandins, Leukotrienes, and Essential Fatty Acids. Nov. 2007;77(5-6):251-261

[62] Cho HP, Nakamura MT, Clarke SD. Cloning, expression, and nutritional regulation of the mammalian Delta-6 desaturase. The Journal of Biological Chemistry. Jan. 1999;**274**(1):471-477

[63] Wang Y, Botolin D, Christian B, Busik J, Xu J, Jump DB. Tissue-specific, nutritional, and developmental regulation of rat fatty acid elongases. Journal of Lipid Research. Apr. 2005;**46**(4):706-715

[64] de Theije CG et al. Dietary long chain n-3 polyunsaturated fatty acids prevent impaired social behaviour and normalize brain dopamine levels in food allergic mice. Neuropharmacology. Mar. 2015;**90**:15-22

[65] Hiratsuka S, Koizumi K, Ooba T, Yokogoshi H. Effects of dietary docosahexaenoic acid connecting phospholipids on the learning ability and fatty acid composition of the brain. Journal of Nutritional Science and Vitaminology (Tokyo). Aug. 2009;**55**(4):374-380

[66] Kitson AP et al. Effect of dietary docosahexaenoic acid (DHA) in phospholipids or triglycerides on brain DHA uptake and accretion. The Journal of Nutritional Biochemistry. Jul. 2016;**33**:91-102

[67] Skorve J et al. Fish oil and krill oil differentially modify the liver and brain lipidome when fed to mice. Lipids in Health and Disease. Aug. 2015;**14**:88

[68] Lacombe RJS, Giuliano V, Colombo SM, Arts MT, Bazinet RP. Compound-specific isotope analysis resolves the dietary origin of docosahexaenoic acid in the mouse brain. Journal of Lipid Research. Oct. 2017;**58**(10):2071-2081

[69] Rey C et al. Dietary n-3 long chain PUFA supplementation promotes a pro-resolving oxylipin profile in the brain. Brain, Behavior, and Immunity. Feb. 2019;**76**:17-27

[70] Orr SK et al. Unesterified docosahexaenoic acid is protective in neuroinflammation. Journal of Neurochemistry. Nov. 2013;**127**(3):378-393

[71] Bascoul-Colombo C, Guschina IA, Maskrey BH, Good M, O'Donnell VB, Harwood JL. Dietary DHA supplementation causes selective changes in phospholipids from different brain regions in both wild type mice and the Tg2576 mouse model of Alzheimer's disease. Biochimica et Biophysica Acta. Jun. 2016;**1861**(6):524-537

[72] Labrousse VF et al. Short-term long chain omega3 diet protects from neuroinflammatory processes and memory impairment in aged mice. PLoS ONE. 2012;7(5):e36861

[73] Boudrault C, Bazinet RP, Kang JX, Ma DW. Cyclooxygenase-2 and n-6 PUFA are lower and DHA is higher in the cortex of fat-1 mice. Neurochemistry International. Mar. 2010;**56**(4):585-589

[74] Bousquet M et al. Transgenic conversion of omega-6 into omega-3 fatty acids in a mouse model of Parkinson's disease. Journal of Lipid Research. Feb. 2011;**52**(2):263-271

[75] He C, Qu X, Cui L, Wang J, Kang JX. Improved spatial learning

performance of fat-1 mice is associated with enhanced neurogenesis and neuritogenesis by docosahexaenoic acid. Proceedings of the National Academy of Sciences of the United States of America. Jul. 2009;**106**(27):11370-11375

[76] Orr SK, Tong JY, Kang JX, Ma DW, Bazinet RP. The fat-1 mouse has brain docosahexaenoic acid levels achievable through fish oil feeding. Neurochemical Research. May 2010;**35**(5):811-819

[77] Delpech J-C et al. Transgenic increase in n-3/n-6 fatty acid ratio protects against cognitive deficits induced by an immune challenge through decrease of neuroinflammation. Neuropsychopharmacology. Feb. 2015;**40**(3):525-536

[78] Bowen RA, Clandinin MT. Maternal dietary 22:6n-3 is more effective than 18nn:3n-3 in increasing the 22:6n-3 content in phospholipids of glial cells from neonatal rat brain. The British Journal of Nutrition. May 2005;**93**(5):601-611

[79] Destaillats F et al. Differential effect of maternal diet supplementation with alpha-linolenic acid or n-3 long-chain polyunsaturated fatty acids on glial cell phosphatidylethanolamine and phosphatidylserine fatty acid profile in neonate rat brains. Nutrition & Metabolism (London). Jan. 2010;7:2

[80] Layé S. Polyunsaturated fatty acids, neuroinflammation and well being. Prostaglandins, Leukotrienes, and Essential Fatty Acids. Jun. 2010;**82**(4-6):295-303

[81] Calder PC. Dietary modification of inflammation with lipids. The Proceedings of the Nutrition Society. Aug. 2002;**61**(3):345-358

[82] Sperling RI, Benincaso AI, Knoell CT, Larkin JK, Austen KF, Robinson DR. Dietary omega-3 polyunsaturated fatty acids inhibit phosphoinositide formation and chemotaxis in neutrophils. The Journal of Clinical Investigation. Feb. 1993;**91**(2):651-660

[83] P. Needleman, A. Raz, M. S. Minkes, J. A. Ferrendelli, and H. Sprecher Triene prostaglandins: Prostacyclin and thromboxane biosynthesis and unique biological properties. Proceedings of the National Academy of Sciences of the United States of America, vol. 76, no. 2, pp. 944-948, Feb. 1979

[84] Obata T, Nagakura T, Masaki T, Maekawa K, Yamashita K. Eicosapentaenoic acid inhibits prostaglandin D2 generation by inhibiting cyclo-oxygenase-2 in cultured human mast cells. Clinical and Experimental Allergy. 1999;**29**(8):1129-1135

[85] Calder PC. n-3 fatty acids, inflammation and immunity: New mechanisms to explain old actions. The Proceedings of the Nutrition Society. Aug. 2013;**72**(3):326-336

[86] Headland SE, Norling LV. The resolution of inflammation: Principles and challenges. Seminars in Immunology. May 2015;**27**(3):149-160

[87] Serhan CN, Chiang N. Resolution phase lipid mediators of inflammation: Agonists of resolution. Current Opinion in Pharmacology. Aug. 2013;**13**(4):632-640

[88] Serhan CN et al. Resolvins: A family of bioactive products of omega-3 fatty acid transformation circuits initiated by aspirin treatment that counter proinflammation signals. The Journal of Experimental Medicine. Oct. 2002;**196**(8):1025-1037

[89] Serhan CN, Chiang N, Van Dyke TE. Resolving inflammation: Dual anti-inflammatory and pro-resolution lipid mediators. Nature Reviews. Immunology. May 2008;**8**(5):349-361

[90] Shalini S-M et al. Distribution of Alox15 in the rat brain and its role in prefrontal cortical resolvin D1 formation and spatial working memory. Molecular Neurobiology. 2018;**55**(2):1537-1550

[91] Nadjar A et al. NFkappaB activates in vivo the synthesis of inducible Cox-2 in the brain. Journal of Cerebral Blood Flow and Metabolism. Aug. 2005;**25**(8):1047-1059

[92] Navarro-Mabarak C, Camacho-Carranza R, Espinosa-Aguirre JJ. Cytochrome P450 in the central nervous system as a therapeutic target in neurodegenerative diseases. Drug Metabolism Reviews. 2018;**50**(2):95-108

[93] Czapski GA, Gajkowska B, Strosznajder JB. Systemic administration of lipopolysaccharide induces molecular and morphological alterations in the hippocampus. Brain Research. Oct. 2010;**1356**:85-94

[94] Schwab JM, Chiang N, Arita M, Serhan CN. Resolvin E1 and protectin D1 activate inflammation-resolution programmes. Nature. Jun. 2007;**447**(7146):869-874

[95] Pratico D et al. 12/15-lipoxygenase is increased in Alzheimer's disease: Possible involvement in brain oxidative stress. The American Journal of Pathology. May 2004;**164**(5):1655-1662

[96] Wang X et al. Resolution of inflammation is altered in Alzheimer's disease. Alzheimer's & Dementia. Jan. 2015;**11**(1):40-50 e1-2

[97] Yigitkanli K, Zheng Y, Pekcec A, Lo EH, van Leyen K. Increased 12/15-lipoxygenase leads to widespread brain injury following global cerebral ischemia. Translational Stroke Research. Apr. 2017;**8**(2):194-202

[98] Sun L, Xu YW, Han J, Liang H, Wang N, Cheng Y. 12/15-Lipoxygenase metabolites of arachidonic acid activate PPARgamma: A possible neuroprotective effect in ischemic brain. Journal of Lipid Research. Mar. 2015;**56**(3):502-514

[99] Bystrom J et al. Endogenous epoxygenases are modulators of monocyte/macrophage activity. PLoS One. 2011;**6**(10):e26591

[100] Fleming I. Cytochrome P450-dependent eicosanoid production and crosstalk. Current Opinion in Lipidology. Oct. 2011;**22**(5):403-409

[101] Gilroy DW et al. CYP450-derived oxylipins mediate inflammatory resolution. Proceedings of the National Academy of Sciences of the United States of America. Jun. 2016;**113**(23):E3240-E3249

[102] Nebert DW, Wikvall K, Miller WL. Human cytochromes P450 in health and disease. Philosophical Transactions of the Royal Society of London. Series B, Biological Sciences. 2013;**368**(1612):20120431

[103] Levi G, Minghetti L, Aloisi F. Regulation of prostanoid synthesis in microglial cells and effects of prostaglandin E2 on microglial functions. Biochimie. Nov. 1998;**80**(11):899-904

[104] Farooqui AA, Horrocks LA, Farooqui T. Modulation of inflammation in brain: A matter of fat. Journal of Neurochemistry. May 2007;**101**(3):577-599

[105] Meyer RP, Gehlhaus M, Knoth R, Volk B. Expression and function of cytochrome p450 in brain drug metabolism. Current Drug Metabolism. May 2007;**8**(4):297-306

[106] Volk B, Hettmannsperger U, Papp T, Amelizad Z, Oesch F, Knoth R. Mapping of phenytoin-inducible cytochrome P450 immunoreactivity

in the mouse central nervous system. Neuroscience. 1991;**42**(1):215-235

[107] Barden AE, Mas E, Mori TA. n-3 Fatty acid supplementation and proresolving mediators of inflammation. Current Opinion in Lipidology. Feb. 2016;**27**(1):26-32

[108] Halade GV, Black LM, Verma MK. Paradigm shift—Metabolic transformation of docosahexaenoic and eicosapentaenoic acids to bioactives exemplify the promise of fatty acid drug discovery. Biotechnology Advances. Aug. 2018;**36**(4):935-953

[109] Recchiuti A. Resolvin D1 and its GPCRs in resolution circuits of inflammation. Prostaglandins & Other Lipid Mediators. Dec. 2013;**107**:64-76

[110] Sun YP et al. Resolvin D1 and its aspirin-triggered 17R epimer. Stereochemical assignments, anti-inflammatory properties, and enzymatic inactivation. The Journal of Biological Chemistry. Mar. 2007;**282**(13):9323-9334

[111] Mulik RS, Bing C, Ladouceur-Wodzak M, Munaweera I, Chopra R, Corbin IR. Localized delivery of low-density lipoprotein docosahexaenoic acid nanoparticles to the rat brain using focused ultrasound. Biomaterials. Mar. 2016;**83**:257-268

[112] Sun W et al. Endogenous expression pattern of resolvin D1 in a rat model of self-resolution of lipopolysaccharide-induced acute respiratory distress syndrome and inflammation. International Immunopharmacology. Nov. 2014;**23**(1):247-253

[113] Bisicchia E et al. Resolvin D1 halts remote neuroinflammation and improves functional recovery after focal brain damage via ALX/FPR2 receptor-regulated microRNAs. Molecular Neurobiology. Aug. 2018;**55**(8):6894-6905

[114] Fredman G, Serhan CN. Specialized proresolving mediator targets for RvE1 and RvD1 in peripheral blood and mechanisms of resolution. The Biochemical Journal. Jul. 2011;**437**(2):185-197

[115] Krishnamoorthy S, Recchiuti A, Chiang N, Fredman G, Serhan CN. Resolvin D1 receptor stereoselectivity and regulation of inflammation and proresolving microRNAs. The American Journal of Pathology. May 2012;**180**(5):2018-2027

[116] Recchiuti A, Krishnamoorthy S, Fredman G, Chiang N, Serhan CN. MicroRNAs in resolution of acute inflammation: Identification of novel resolvin D1-miRNA circuits. The FASEB Journal. Feb. 2011;**25**(2):544-560

[117] Rey C et al. Resolvin D1 and E1 promote resolution of inflammation in microglial cells in vitro. Brain, Behavior, and Immunity. Jul. 2016;**55**:249-259

[118] Aursnes M et al. Total synthesis of the lipid mediator PD1n-3 DPA: Configurational assignments and anti-inflammatory and pro-resolving actions. Journal of Natural Products. Apr. 2014;77(4):910-916

[119] Doyle R, Sadlier DM, Godson C. Pro-resolving lipid mediators: Agents of anti-ageing? Seminars in Immunology. 2018;**40**:36-48

[120] Hong S, Gronert K, Devchand PR, Moussignac RL, Serhan CN. Novel docosatrienes and 17S-resolvins generated from docosahexaenoic acid in murine brain, human blood, and glial cells. Autacoids in anti-inflammation. The Journal of Biological Chemistry. 2003;**278**(17):14677-14687

[121] Kuda O. Bioactive metabolites of docosahexaenoic acid. Biochimie. May 2017;**136**:12-20

[122] Marcheselli VL et al. Novel docosanoids inhibit brain

ischemia-reperfusion-mediated leukocyte infiltration and pro-inflammatory gene expression. The Journal of Biological Chemistry. Oct. 2003;**278**(44):43807-43817

[123] Lukiw WJ et al. A role for docosahexaenoic acid-derived neuroprotectin D1 in neural cell survival and Alzheimer disease. The Journal of Clinical Investigation. Oct. 2005;**115**(10):2774-2783

[124] Bazan NG et al. Novel aspirin-triggered neuroprotectin D1 attenuates cerebral ischemic injury after experimental stroke. Experimental Neurology. Jul. 2012;**236**(1):122-130

[125] Yao C, Zhang J, Chen F, Lin Y. Neuroprotectin D1 attenuates brain damage induced by transient middle cerebral artery occlusion in rats through TRPC6/CREB pathways. Molecular Medicine Reports. Aug. 2013;**8**(2):543-550

[126] Serhan CN et al. Maresins: Novel macrophage mediators with potent antiinflammatory and proresolving actions. The Journal of Experimental Medicine. Jan. 2009;**206**(1):15-23

[127] Zhu M et al. Pro-resolving lipid mediators improve neuronal survival and increase Abeta42 phagocytosis. Molecular Neurobiology. May 2016;**53**(4):2733-2749

[128] Xian W et al. The pro-resolving lipid mediator Maresin 1 protects against cerebral ischemia/reperfusion injury by attenuating the pro-inflammatory response. Biochemical and Biophysical Research Communications. Mar. 2016;**472**(1):175-181

[129] Xian W, Li T, Li L, Hu L, Cao J. Maresin 1 attenuates the inflammatory response and mitochondrial damage in mice with cerebral ischemia/reperfusion in a SIRT1-dependent manner. Brain Research. 2019

[130] Francos-Quijorna I et al. Maresin 1 promotes inflammatory resolution, neuroprotection, and functional neurological recovery after spinal cord injury. The Journal of Neuroscience. Nov. 2017;**37**(48):11731-11743

[131] Ohira T, Arita M, Omori K, Recchiuti A, Van Dyke TE, Serhan CN. Resolvin E1 receptor activation signals phosphorylation and phagocytosis. The Journal of Biological Chemistry. Jan. 2010;**285**(5):3451-3461

[132] Isobe Y et al. Identification and structure determination of novel anti-inflammatory mediator resolvin E3, 17,18-dihydroxyeicosapentaenoic acid. The Journal of Biological Chemistry. Mar. 2012;**287**(13):10525-10534

[133] Chen CT, Liu Z, Bazinet RP. Rapid de-esterification and loss of eicosapentaenoic acid from rat brain phospholipids: An intracerebroventricular study. Journal of Neurochemistry. Feb. 2011;**116**(3):363-373

[134] Siegert E, Paul F, Rothe M, Weylandt KH. The effect of omega-3 fatty acids on central nervous system remyelination in fat-1 mice. BMC Neuroscience. 2017;**18**(1):19

[135] Krishnamoorthy S et al. Resolvin D1 binds human phagocytes with evidence for proresolving receptors. Proceedings of the National Academy of Sciences of the United States of America. Jan. 2010;**107**(4):1660-1665

[136] Arita M, Ohira T, Sun YP, Elangovan S, Chiang N, Serhan CN. Resolvin E1 selectively interacts with leukotriene B4 receptor BLT1 and ChemR23 to regulate inflammation. Journal of Immunology. Mar. 2007;**178**(6):3912-3917

[137] Ho CF-Y et al. Localisation of formyl-peptide receptor 2 in the rat central nervous system and its role in axonal and dendritic outgrowth. Neurochemical Research. Aug. 2018;**43**(8):1587-1598

[138] Guo X et al. Chronic mild restraint stress rats decreased CMKLR1 expression in distinct brain region. Neuroscience Letters. Aug. 2012;**524**(1):25-29

[139] Graham KL et al. Chemokine-like receptor-1 expression by central nervous system-infiltrating leukocytes and involvement in a model of autoimmune demyelinating disease. Journal of Immunology. 2009;**183**(10):6717-6723

[140] Xu ZZ et al. Resolvins RvE1 and RvD1 attenuate inflammatory pain via central and peripheral actions. Nature Medicine. May 2010;**16**(5):592-597, 1p following 597

[141] Qu L, Caterina MJ. Accelerating the reversal of inflammatory pain with NPD1 and its receptor GPR37. The Journal of Clinical Investigation. Aug. 2018;**128**(8):3246-3249

[142] Colas RA, Shinohara M, Dalli J, Chiang N, Serhan CN. Identification and signature profiles for pro-resolving and inflammatory lipid mediators in human tissue. American Journal of Physiology-Cell Physiology. Jul. 2014;**307**(1):C39-C54

[143] Serhan CN, Chiang N, Dalli J. New pro-resolving n-3 mediators bridge resolution of infectious inflammation to tissue regeneration. Molecular Aspects of Medicine. Dec. 2018;**64**:1-17

[144] Famenini S et al. Increased intermediate M1-M2 macrophage polarization and improved cognition in mild cognitive impairment patients on omega-3 supplementation. The FASEB Journal. Jan. 2017;**31**(1):148-160

[145] Mizwicki MT et al. 1alpha,25-dihydroxyvitamin D3 and resolvin D1 retune the balance between amyloid-beta phagocytosis and inflammation in Alzheimer's disease patients. Journal of Alzheimer's Disease. 2013;**34**(1):155-170

[146] Uno H et al. Immunonutrition suppresses acute inflammatory responses through modulation of resolvin E1 in patients undergoing major hepatobiliary resection. Surgery. 2016;**160**(1):228-236

[147] Hiram R et al. Resolvin E1 normalizes contractility, Ca^{2+} sensitivity and smooth muscle cell migration rate in TNF-α- and IL-6-pretreated human pulmonary arteries. American Journal of Physiology. Lung Cellular and Molecular Physiology. Oct. 2015;**309**(8):L776-L788

[148] Gyurko R, Van Dyke TE. The role of polyunsaturated ω-3 fatty acid eicosapentaenoic acid-derived resolvin E1 (RvE1) in bone preservation. Critical Reviews in Immunology. 2014;**34**(4):347-357

[149] Abdelmoaty S et al. Spinal actions of lipoxin A4 and 17(R)-resolvin D1 attenuate inflammation-induced mechanical hypersensitivity and spinal TNF release. PLoS One. 2013;**8**(9):e75543

[150] Rossi S et al. Protection from endotoxic uveitis by intravitreal resolvin D1: Involvement of lymphocytes, miRNAs, ubiquitin-proteasome, and M1/M2 macrophages. Mediators of Inflammation. 2015;**2015**:149381

[151] Titos E et al. Resolvin D1 and its precursor docosahexaenoic acid promote resolution of adipose tissue inflammation by eliciting macrophage polarization toward an M2-like phenotype. Journal of Immunology. Nov. 2011;**187**(10):5408-5418

[152] Li L et al. Resolvin D1 promotes the interleukin-4-induced alternative activation in BV-2 microglial cells. Journal of Neuroinflammation. 2014;**11**:72

[153] Kantarci A et al. Combined administration of resolvin E1 and lipoxin A4 resolves inflammation in a murine model of Alzheimer's disease. Experimental Neurology. 2018;**300**:111-120

[154] Harrison JL et al. Resolvins AT-D1 and E1 differentially impact functional outcome, post-traumatic sleep, and microglial activation following diffuse brain injury in the mouse. Brain, Behavior, and Immunity. Jul. 2015;**47**:131-140

[155] Xu MX et al. Resolvin D1, an endogenous lipid mediator for inactivation of inflammation-related signaling pathways in microglial cells, prevents lipopolysaccharide-induced inflammatory responses. CNS Neuroscience & Therapeutics. Apr. 2013;**19**(4):235-243

[156] Terrando N et al. Aspirin-triggered resolvin D1 prevents surgery-induced cognitive decline. The FASEB Journal. Sep. 2013;**27**(9):3564-3571

[157] Luo C et al. Enriched endogenous omega-3 fatty acids in mice protect against global ischemia injury. Journal of Lipid Research. Jul. 2014;**55**(7):1288-1297

[158] Furuyashiki T, Akiyama S, Kitaoka S. Roles of multiple lipid mediators in stress and depression. International Immunology. 2019

[159] Deyama S et al. Resolvin D1 and D2 reverse lipopolysaccharide-induced depression-like behaviors through the mTORC1 signaling pathway. The International Journal of Neuropsychopharmacology. Jul. 2017;**20**(7):575-584

[160] Deyama S et al. Resolvin E1/E2 ameliorate lipopolysaccharide-induced depression-like behaviors via ChemR23. Psychopharmacology. 2018;**235**(1):329-336

[161] Deyama S, Shimoda K, Ikeda H, Fukuda H, Shuto S, Minami M. Resolvin E3 attenuates lipopolysaccharide-induced depression-like behavior in mice. Journal of Pharmacological Sciences. Sep. 2018;**138**(1):86-88

[162] Klein CP, Sperotto ND, Maciel IS, Leite CE, Souza AH, Campos MM. Effects of D-series resolvins on behavioral and neurochemical changes in a fibromyalgia-like model in mice. Neuropharmacology. Nov. 2014;**86**:57-66

[163] Gilbert K, Bernier J, Godbout R, Rousseau G. Resolvin D1, a metabolite of omega-3 polyunsaturated fatty acid, decreases post-myocardial infarct depression. Marine Drugs. Nov. 2014;**12**(11):5396-5407

[164] Ishikawa Y et al. Rapid and sustained antidepressant effects of resolvin D1 and D2 in a chronic unpredictable stress model. Behavioural Brain Research. Aug. 2017;**332**:233-236

[165] Zhu M, Wang X, Schultzberg M, Hjorth E. Differential regulation of resolution in inflammation induced by amyloid-β42 and lipopolysaccharides in human microglia. Journal of Alzheimer's Disease. 2015;**43**(4):1237-1250

[166] Tian Y, Zhang Y, Zhang R, Qiao S, Fan J. Resolvin D2 recovers neural injury by suppressing inflammatory mediators expression in lipopolysaccharide-induced Parkinson's disease rat model. Biochemical and Biophysical Research Communications. May 2015;**460**(3):799-805

[167] Shevalye H et al. Effect of enriching the diet with menhaden oil or daily treatment with resolvin D1 on

neuropathy in a mouse model of type 2 diabetes. Journal of Neurophysiology. Jul. 2015;**114**(1):199-208

[168] Hashimoto M et al. n-3 fatty acids effectively improve the reference memory-related learning ability associated with increased brain docosahexaenoic acid-derived docosanoids in aged rats. Biochimica et Biophysica Acta. Feb. 2015;**1851**(2):203-209

[169] Taha AY et al. Regulation of rat plasma and cerebral cortex oxylipin concentrations with increasing levels of dietary linoleic acid. Prostaglandins, Leukotrienes & Essential Fatty Acids. 2016

[170] Ostermann AI et al. A diet rich in omega-3 fatty acids enhances expression of soluble epoxide hydrolase in murine brain. Prostaglandins & Other Lipid Mediators. Nov. 2017;**133**:79-87

[171] Farias SE, Basselin M, Chang L, Heidenreich KA, Rapoport SI, Murphy RC. Formation of eicosanoids, E2/D2 isoprostanes, and docosanoids following decapitation-induced ischemia, measured in high-energy-microwaved rat brain. Journal of Lipid Research. Sep. 2008;**49**(9):1990-2000

[172] Yang G, Pan F, Gan WB. Stably maintained dendritic spines are associated with lifelong memories. Nature. Dec. 2009;**462**(7275):920-924

[173] Balvers MG et al. Fish oil and inflammatory status alter the n-3 to n-6 balance of the endocannabinoid and oxylipin metabolomes in mouse plasma and tissues. Metabolomics. Dec. 2012;**8**(6):1130-1147

[174] Willenberg I, Rund K, Rong S, Shushakova N, Gueler F, Schebb NH. Characterization of changes in plasma and tissue oxylipin levels in LPS and CLP induced murine sepsis. Inflammation Research. Feb. 2016;**65**(2):133-142

[175] Rosenberger TA et al. Rat brain arachidonic acid metabolism is increased by a 6-day intracerebral ventricular infusion of bacterial lipopolysaccharide. Journal of Neurochemistry. Mar. 2004;**88**(5):1168-1178

[176] Taha AY et al. Dietary linoleic acid lowering reduces lipopolysaccharide-induced increase in brain arachidonic acid metabolism. Molecular Neurobiology. Aug. 2017;**54**(6):4303-4315

[177] Dieter P, Scheibe R, Kamionka S, Kolada A. LPS-induced synthesis and release of PGE2 in liver macrophages: Regulation by CPLA2, COX-1, COX-2, and PGE2 synthase. Advances in Experimental Medicine and Biology. 2002;**507**:457-462

[178] Le Faouder P et al. LC-MS/MS method for rapid and concomitant quantification of pro-inflammatory and pro-resolving polyunsaturated fatty acid metabolites. Journal of Chromatography. B, Analytical Technologies in the Biomedical and Life Sciences. Aug. 2013;**932**:123-133

[179] Slepko N, Minghetti L, Polazzi E, Nicolini A, Levi G. Reorientation of prostanoid production accompanies 'activation' of adult microglial cells in culture. Journal of Neuroscience Research. Aug. 1997;**49**(3):292-300

[180] Wang C, Wang M, Zhou Y, Dupree JL, Han X. Alterations in mouse brain lipidome after disruption of CST gene: A lipidomics study. Molecular Neurobiology. Aug. 2014;**50**(1):88-96

[181] Jung YS et al. Probucol inhibits LPS-induced microglia activation and ameliorates brain ischemic injury in normal and hyperlipidemic mice. Acta Pharmacologica Sinica. Aug. 2016;**37**(8):1031-1044

[182] Kim HW, Rao JS, Rapoport SI, Igarashi M. Dietary n-6 PUFA deprivation downregulates arachidonate but upregulates docosahexaenoate metabolizing enzymes in rat brain. Biochimica et Biophysica Acta. Feb. 2011;**1811**(2):111-117

Section 3

Carbohydrates and the Brain

Chapter 3

Carbohydrates and the Brain: Roles and Impact

Xavier Fioramonti and Luc Pénicaud

Abstract

Even if its size is fairly small (about 2% of body weight), the brain consumes around 20% of the total body energy. Whereas organs such as muscles and liver may use several sources of energy, under physiological conditions, the brain mainly depends on glucose for its energy needs. This involves the need for blood glucose level to be tightly regulated. Thus, in addition to its fueling role, glucose plays a role as signaling molecule informing the brain of any slight change in blood level to ensure glucose homeostasis. In this chapter, we will describe the fueling and sensing properties of glucose and other carbohydrates on the brain and present some physiological brain functions impacted by these sugars. We will also highlight the scientific questions that need to be answered in order to better understand the impact of sugars on the brain.

Keywords: brain, glucose, fructose, food intake, glucose-sensing neurons

1. Introduction

The mammalian brain essentially depends on glucose for its energy needs. Because neurons have the highest energy demand in the adult brain, they require continuous delivery of glucose from the blood. In man, the brain represents ~2% of the body weight but uses ~20% of glucose-derived energy, making it the main consumer of glucose [1]. As a consequence, a tight regulation of glucose metabolism is critical for brain physiology. A fine feedback loop between the brain and various organs and tissues has been demonstrated, allowing, in normal conditions, to maintain blood glucose level rather constant around 1 g/l (7–8 mM) in the blood and ~2 mM in the brain (see below Section 5) [2, 3]. The brain needs a precise and clear feedback on the metabolic state of the whole body [4]. To achieve this aim, various brain areas, especially the brainstem and the hypothalamus, integrate peripheral signals delivered by neural input from various organs, as well as by metabolites (glucose, fatty acids) and hormones (leptin, insulin, ghrelin) via the blood [2–4]. Thus, specialized nutrients- and hormones-sensing neurons in which the firing rate varies in response to changes in extra-cellular nutrients or hormones concentration have been described. In response, the brain will generate appropriate response by modulating food intake and peripheral organs' activity via the autonomic nervous system to maintain energy status and glucose homeostasis (**Figure 1**). Thus, we will describe in this chapter that in the central nervous system, glucose has a dual role and is considered as a fueling as well as a sensing metabolite to ensure glucose homeostasis and appropriate fueling of brain cells.

IntechOpen

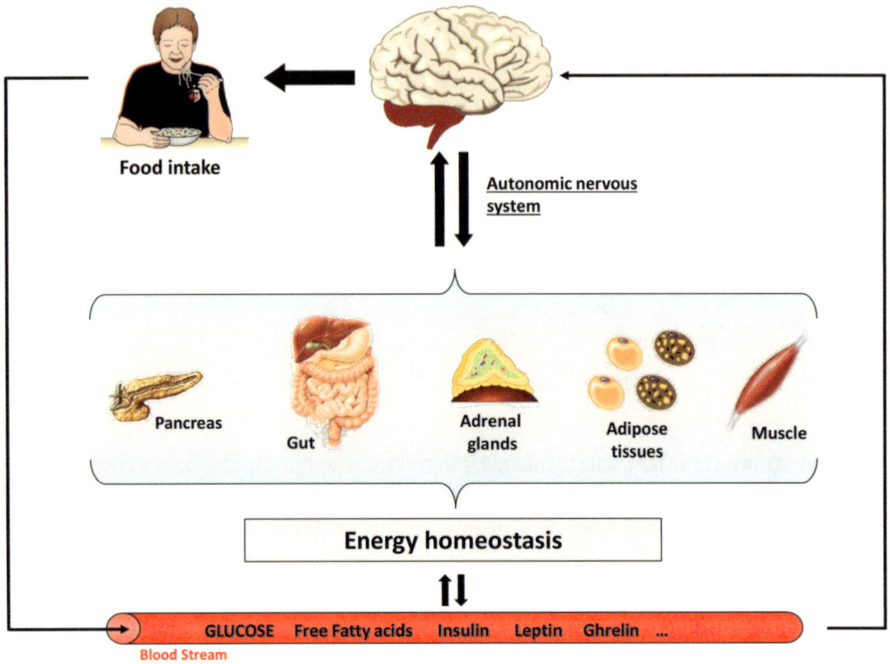

Figure 1.
Role of the brain in the control of energy homeostasis. The brain integrates peripheral signals delivered by neural input from various organs, as well as by metabolites (glucose and fatty acids) and hormones (leptin, insulin, and ghrelin) via the blood. In response, the brain generates appropriate response by modulating food intake and peripheral organs' activity via the autonomic nervous system to maintain energy homeostasis.

However, one has to keep in mind that given the dietary mutations that occurred in recent decades, sugars other than glucose are part of our diet and could influence brain fueling and sensing. This is indeed the case for example of fructose. Fructose and glucose are rather simple molecules but there are differences in the way the body processes them. This is definitely true for the way the brain uses and reacts to them. These differences could explain the consequences observed after a high consumption of fructose, on food intake and whole-body glucose metabolism.

2. Brain's control of glycemia

In humans, the value for normoglycemia is around 1 g/l. Although the endocrine pancreas is the main regulator of blood glucose level via the secretion of insulin and glucagon, the brain plays a major role in controlling glycemia. This is achieved through different pathways involving the autonomic nervous system and its projection to several organs and tissues such as the endocrine pancreas, the adrenal gland, the liver, skeletal muscles, and white and brown adipose tissues. As illustrated in **Figure 2**, in case of a drop in blood glucose, there is an activation of sympathetic nerves and consequently an increase in glucagon secretion by the alpha cells and a decrease in that of insulin by the beta cells of the pancreas, as well as an increase in epinephrine and cortisol secretion by the adrenal gland. These changes in hormone levels together with a direct effect of the sympathetic system will lead to an increased glucose production by the liver, and a decreased glucose utilization by fat deposits and muscles, leading thus to a normalization of blood glucose.

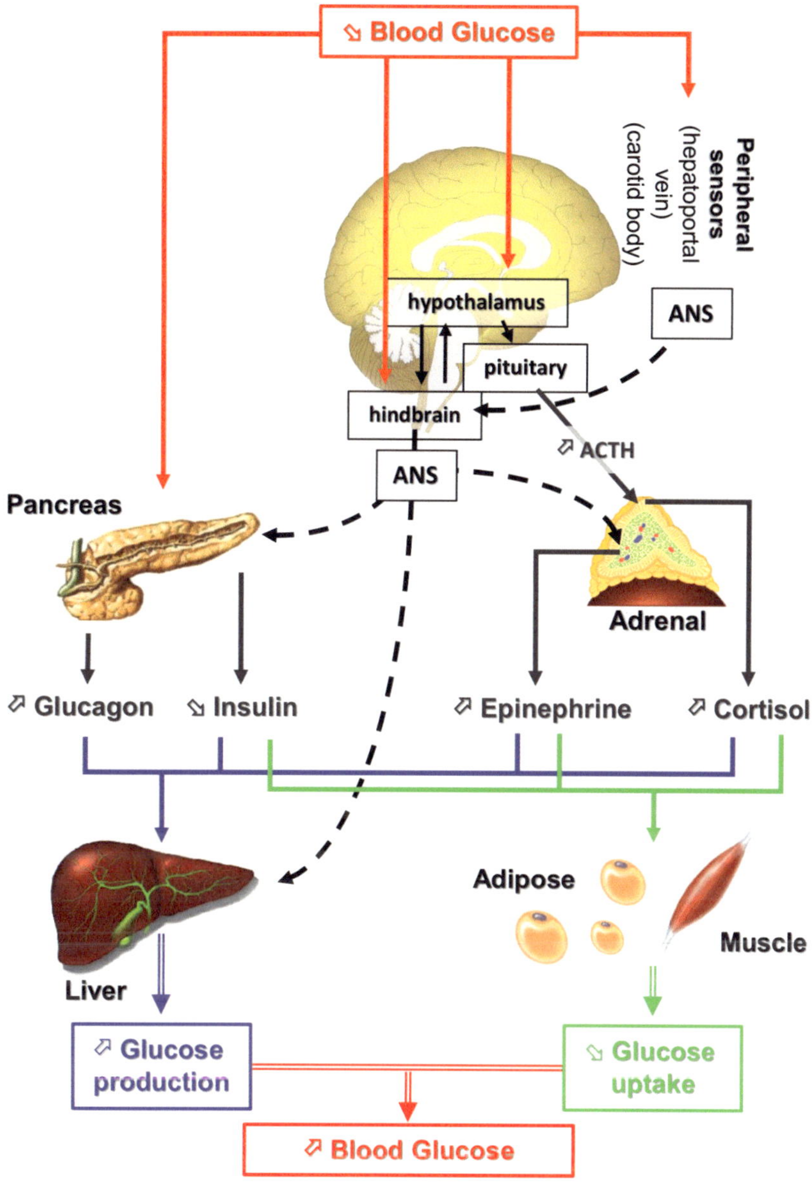

Figure 2.
Neuroendocrine pathways involved in the counter-regulatory response to hypoglycemia. Decreased blood glucose is detected by central (hypothalamus and hindbrain) and peripheral (pancreas, hepatoportal vein, and carotid body) glucose sensors. Together, these glucose sensors coordinate physiological responses, which raise blood glucose levels. The initial response to hypoglycemia involves activation of the autonomic nervous system (ANS), inhibition of insulin secretion, and stimulation of pituitary ACTH secretion. Activation of the autonomic nervous system increases glucagon and epinephrine secretion from the pancreas and adrenal medulla, respectively. ACTH stimulates cortisol release from the adrenal cortex. Increased glucagon, epinephrine, and cortisol together with decreased insulin stimulate hepatic glucose production and decrease adipose and muscle glucose uptake. The net result of the neuroendocrine counter-regulatory response to hypoglycemia is to increase blood glucose levels and restore euglycemia.

3. Glucose: the fuel of brain's neurons

Brain function and glucose metabolism are intimately linked [1]. Indeed, glucose is the main, if not the only, energy substrate of this organ. Hypoglycemia (below 0.7 g/l) causes rapid brain repercussions, but fortunately, most of the time quickly reversible after correction of hypoglycemia. With regard to hyperglycemia, acute situations such as ketoacidosis and hyperosmolarity can lead to a coma, with significant mortality. The chronic effects of hyperglycemia on the brain remain unclear, apart from the risk of ischemic stroke. However, microangiopathy is intimately linked to chronic hyperglycemia, and can cause irreversible diffuse vascular lesions and cerebral ischemia, resulting in cortical atrophy and diabetic encephalopathy.

The brain uses glucose as its main source of energy, although it can utilize other metabolites (mainly ketone bodies) in special situations such as fasting. It has very high energy consumption for its size, mainly due to the high energy supply needed to maintain its functions (potential difference across nerve cell membranes, transport along axons and dendrites, tissue plasticity and repair).

Glucose enters the brain by facilitated diffusion across the blood-brain barrier, and enters brain cells mainly via a range of glucose transporters. Most human cells import glucose by members of the GLUT (SLC2A) family of membrane transport proteins (see review [5]). Of these, GLUT1 is abundant at the BBB and in astrocytes, regulated mainly by steady-state levels of plasma glucose. GLUT2 appears to serve glucose sensors in the brain. GLUT3 ensures efficient glucose uptake by neurons. Although the brain is considered as a non-insulin-dependent organ, insulin crosses the blood-brain barrier and binds to receptors on neurons and glial cells [6]. There is controversy as to whether insulin resistance for glucose is present in the CNS, but emerging data suggest that insulin insensitivity may play an important role in the pathogenesis of obesity, type 2 diabetes, and Alzheimer's disease [7, 8]. GLUT5 and GLUT7 are present at low levels in the brain and have specificity for fructose. GLUT6 is expressed in the brain but has low affinity to glucose. Studies of mice suggest roles of GLUT8 in hippocampal neuronal proliferation. GLUT13 is a myoinositol transporter expressed primarily in the brain and is the only GLUT protein that appears to function as a proton-coupled symporter (see review [5]).

Once transported into the cell, glucose is phosphorylated by a hexokinase, an enzyme with such high affinity toward glucose that it rapidly transforms glucose into glucose-6-phosphate. Glucose-6-phosphate is metabolized further, mainly in the glycolytic pathway, where it is converted to pyruvate. Glucose-6-phosphate is also substrate for the pentose phosphate shunt and the generation of glycogen only in glial cells. Pyruvate is metabolized either in the Krebs cycle after transport into the mitochondria, or converted to lactate by means of the lactate dehydrogenase. A large part of the pyruvate transported into brain mitochondria is devoted to the oxidative phosphorylation of ADP to ATP.

The energy supply to the brain is provided by blood vessels. In most brain structures, these vessels are surrounded by a blood-brain barrier which does not allow molecules to cross it and as a consequence isolates the brain from the circulatory network. Under these conditions, the energy input is partly indirect and passes partly through the cells that constitute this barrier, namely the astrocytes [9]. These cells can store energy as glycogen or transform it as lactate. This energy is released on demand, when the neurons need it [10]. This lactate is produced in astrocytes by degradation of glucose in pyruvate when the neurons need it. The lactate is then sent to neurons, which synthetize pyruvate and use it in the Krebs cycle. This role of astrocytes and lactate as the main energy substrate of neurons is still a matter of debates.

4. Glucose: a signaling molecule for the brain

In the previous part, we discussed the fact that the brain relies on glucose to function. This implies that blood glucose level must remain stable. Any decrease in blood glucose level would have immediate consequences on brain functions. Increased blood level will not have acute consequences but sustained hyperglycemia will be deleterious in the long term as seen in patients with uncontrolled diabetes mellitus. The brain plays a critical role in the regulation of blood glucose level to ensure whole-body glucose homeostasis. Thus, to be able to control the level of blood glucose, the brain must be able to sense any change. In this part, we will discuss the idea that glucose is more than a fueling molecule and it is able to play the role of a signaling molecule in some neurons or brain cells called glucose-sensing cells.

Glucose-sensing neurons: The first hypothesis that specialized cells within the brain could detect changes in glucose level originated from studies by Oomura' and Anand's groups, in which they showed that neurons within the hypothalamus had their electrical activity modified in response to intravenous injection of glucose [11, 12]. While these studies suggested that neurons able to detect glucose were present in the brain, they did not prove that glucose could directly affect these neurons since glucose was injected intravenously. Thus, later, Oomura demonstrated the presence of specialized glucose-sensing neurons in showing that the direct application of glucose in the lateral hypothalamus of rats altered the activity of specific neurons [13]. These so-called glucose-sensing neurons are now defined as cells able to adapt their electrical activity in response to changes in extracellular glucose level. By definition, glucose-excited (GE) neurons increase their electrical activity, whereas glucose-inhibited (GI) neurons decrease their activity when glucose level rises. By opposition, when glucose level decreases, GE neurons decrease their electrical activity whereas GI neurons increase it (**Figure 3**).

It is important to note that glucose-sensing neurons use glucose, not only as fuel, but as a signaling molecule that modulates their electrical activity. In addition, it must be mentioned that glucose-sensing neurons directly detect changes in glucose level and not through indirect presynaptic modulation. Finally, their responses to decreased glucose level are distinct from the "run-out-of-fuel" silencing of every neuron by nonphysiological low glucose levels.

Brain glucose level: The notion that, by definition, glucose-sensing neurons respond to physiological changes in brain glucose level raises the question of the

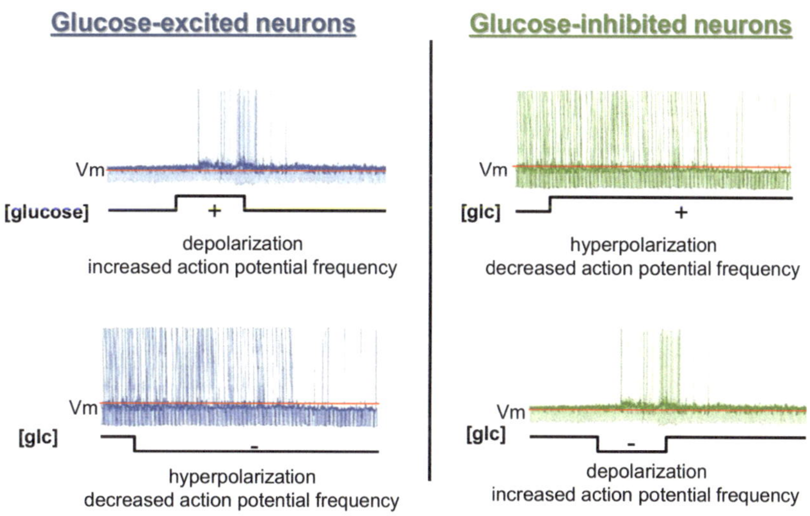

Figure 3.
Schematic representation of the electrical activity of glucose-sensing neurons in response to changes in glucose level. Glucose-excited (GE) neurons increase their electrical activity (depolarization and increased action potential frequency), whereas glucose-inhibited (GI) neurons decrease their activity (hyperpolarization and decreased firing rate) when glucose level rises. By opposition, when glucose level decreases, GE neurons decrease their electrical activity whereas GI neurons increase it. Abbreviations: glucose or glc, extracellular glucose level; Vm, basal membrane potential.

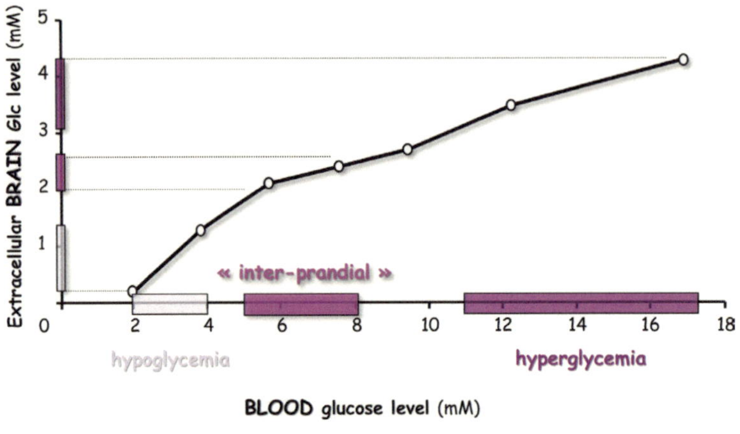

Figure 4.
Extracellular brain glucose levels versus plasma glucose levels. Plasma glucose levels of about 2–4 mM (50–80 mg/dl) observed during hypoglycemia correlate brain levels of about 0.1–1 mM. Plasma levels of about 5–8 (80–120 mg/dl) are related to levels seen during meal-to-meal variation and correlate to brain levels of about 2–2.5 mM. Plasma glucose levels over 8 mM or 140 mg/dl are seen during uncontrolled hyperglycemia and correlate with brain level above 3 mM but not exceeding 4.5–5 mM. Adapted from Ref. [19].

glucose level in the brain. The level of brain glucose is a process finely regulated by GLUT1, the glucose transporter expressed at the BBB. The high affinity of this transporter (K_M = 2–3 mM) for glucose justifies the level found in the brain, which is about 30% of the blood level. Thus, several studies using glucose oxidase electrode methods or zero net flux method for microdialysis consistently indicate that physiological levels of glucose within the brain vary within a fairly tight range from 0.7 to 2.5 mM. On the other hand, extracellular brain glucose levels below 0.7 mM and above 2.5 mM are associated pathological hypo- and hyperglycemia, respectively. This is the case in all brain areas where it has been measured including the hypothalamus, the hippocampus, and striatum for instance [14–18] (**Figure 4**).

Location and role of glucose-sensing neurons: Most of the glucose-sensing neurons have been described in the hypothalamus in response to changes in the window between 0.1 and 5 mM, which represents the physiological changes observed in the brain (see for review [20, 21]). Nevertheless, our group found that within the arcuate nucleus (ARC), four populations of glucose-sensing neurons actually exist. We showed that the "classical" GE and GI neurons detect changes below 2.5 mM whereas so-called HGE or HGI neurons (for high-glucose-excited or -inhibited neurons) are respectively activated or inhibited by changes above 5 mM [22–25]. Interestingly, the electrical activity of HGE and HGI neurons is only changed in response to glucose change below 2.5 mM and not altered by changes in glucose level above it [22, 23]. Similarly, we found that HGE and HGI neurons only change their electrical activity in response to changes in glucose level above 5 mM but not below this level [23]. Finding these different subpopulations of glucose-sensing neurons raised the question of the actual glucose level present in the arcuate nucleus of the hypothalamus in which the BBB is fenestrated [16, 26] and suggested that, in confined areas, glucose level could be increased closer to levels found in the blood.

Not everything is known yet regarding these different populations of glucose-sensing neurons. Their proportion within the different nuclei of the hypothalamus is difficult to estimate since not every study uses the same changes in glucose level. However, we could estimate that they represent around 10% of hypothalamic neurons. A question which has been poorly addressed is their interconnection. We think that some HGE or HGI neurons from the ARC may connect some VMN neurons found to be indirectly modulated to increased glucose level above

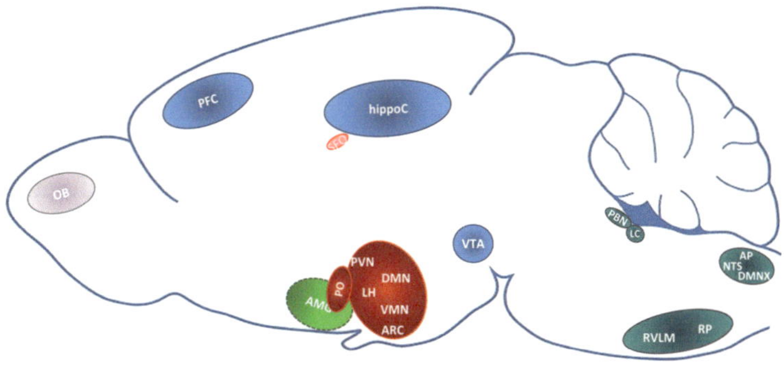

Figure 5.
Location of brain glucose-sensing neurons. Schematic representation of a sagittal slice of a rodent brain with different areas where glucose-sensing neurons have been found. Abbreviations: AMG, amygdala; AP, area postrema; ARC, arcuate nucleus; DMNX, dorsal motor nucleus; DMN, dorsomedial nucleus; HippoC, hippocampus; LC, locus coeruleus; LH, lateral hypothalamus; NTS, solitary nucleus; OB, olfactory bulb; PBN, parabrachial nucleus; PFC, prefrontal cortex; PO, preoptic area; PVN, paraventricular nucleus; RP, Raphe pallidus; SFO, subfornical organ; VMN, ventromedial nucleus; VTA, ventral tegmental area.

5 mM [20, 23, 27]. Nevertheless, no study has directly studied their interconnection to determine whether they could work as a synchronous network. By opposition, the molecular mechanisms involved in their detection to changes in glucose level are pretty much known (see for review [20, 21]). The nature of these glucose-sensing neurons in terms of neurotransmitter expressed and released, however, is not clear for all the subpopulations [20]. Knowing better the identity of glucose-sensing neurons will be necessary to better understand the physiological functions they control, which are not fully understood yet. It is however clear that these neurons are involved in the control of food intake, thermogenesis, and glucose homeostasis (glucose tolerance, insulin secretion, and hepatic glucose production). Several studies have described that inhibiting molecular mechanisms involved in their glucose sensitivity alters some of these functions.

Glucose-sensing neurons can be found in extra-hypothalamic areas (**Figure** 5). To our knowledge, HGE and HGI neurons have only been found in so-called circumventricular organs, brain areas where the BBB is fenestrated including the area postrema of the hindbrain, the subfornical organ and the vascular organ of lamina terminalis. All the other brain areas where glucose-sensing have been found present neurons modulated by glucose changes below 2.5 mM glucose. This raises the question of the physiological role of these neurons in these extra-hypothalamic areas. One hypothesis is that these neurons present in different places of the brain detect decreased glucose level, which could be associated to hypoglycemia. They may play the role of detectors of energy availability and inform about a potential "crisis" since glucose is the principal fuel of neurons and its brain level needs to be finely controlled. Nevertheless, we cannot exclude that these neurons take part in physiological functions including memory, motivation olfaction, in view of their location in areas such as the hippocampus, striatum, olfactory bulb for instance. Significant work is still needed to fully understand the functions controlled by these hypothalamic or extra-hypothalamic neurons.

Glial cells are also able to detect glucose: Astrocytes represent the major class of macroglial brain cells and occupy about 50% of the total brain volume. Beyond their role of structural neuronal supporting cells, astrocytes are now recognized to take an acting part in brain homeostasis and participate in increasingly large number of functions including neuronal proliferation, synaptogenesis, synaptic transmission, and neurotransmitter homeostasis as well as neuronal fueling and nutrient sensing.

The first evidence suggesting a role of astrocytes in hypothalamic glucose-sensing was the expression of some key "glucose-sensing" protein in this cell population. Thus, our group was the first to show that GLUT2 is expressed in hypothalamic astrocytes [28–30]. Other glucose sensors such as K_{ATP} channels and glucokinase are also found in astrocytes. We also showed that increased central glucose level increases the expression of the cell activation maker c-fos in hypothalamic astrocytes [31]. More recently, studies showed that glial cells are directly glucose-sensing using primary culture. Thus, increased glucose level increases calcium waves in hypothalamic tanycytes (astrocyte-like cells present in the ventral hypothalamus) suggesting that these cells are activated by glucose as shown in neurons [32, 33]. Even though these studies started to decipher mechanisms involved in astrocyte glucose-sensing (involvement of ATP release, purinergic channels, connexins), further work is still needed to better understand the signaling pathways involved in their glucose-sensing. A question that needs to be answered is the mechanisms by which astrocytes and neurons are coupled in order to ensure brain glucose-sensing. Studies from our group and others suggested that the gliotransmitter ACBP (AcetylCoA-Binding Protein), released by astrocytes in response to increased glucose level, activates pro-opiomelanocortin neurons of the arcuate nucleus, neurons highly known to control food intake, thermogenesis, and glucose homeostasis [34, 35]. ACBP is not the only gliotransmitter involved in glucose-sensing, other studies also showed the importance of ATP or lactate. Interestingly, glucose-excited neurons responding to increased glucose level are also activated by lactate [36]. Thus, in addition to be a fueling substrate for neurons, lactate, as glucose, is also considered as a signaling-like nutrient for glucose-sensing neurons. More studies are still needed to highlight other potential glucose-sensing gliotransmitter and to fully understand the role of astrocytes in brain glucose-sensing. Also, different isoforms of glucose transporters or hexokinases are expressed in other glial cells including microglia or oligodendrocytes [37]. Nevertheless, except a putative fueling role, it is not known whether these glial cell types are able to sense changes in glucose levels as neurons or astrocytes do.

5. The impact of other sugars on the brain: the example of fructose

The patterns of sugar consumption have changed considerably in recent decades. Glucose is not the only monosaccharide present in our alimentation, which can cross the intestinal barrier and be present in the bloodstream. Fructose is the other main monosaccharide we eat. Fructose is the *partner* of glucose in the sucrose we consume. In addition to its natural presence in fruit and honey, it is also present in soda, biscuits, and all sorts of processed food. Thus, while fructose consumption was <5 g/day until the 70s, it consumption has dramatically increased since and currently reaches 50–80 g/day in developed countries. In addition, the ending of European sugar quota in 2017 will likely further increase by 8–15% its intake in the next decade.

So far, the increase in fructose consumption has raised health issues regarding liver function and development of metabolic syndrome [38]. Increases in fructose consumption have paralleled the increasing prevalence of obesity, and high-fructose diets are thought to promote weight gain and insulin resistance. Thus, fructose has been pointed out by the French Anses agency as potentially harmful (saisine n° 2012-SA-0186). The agency demands "more studies aiming at understanding the effect of selective sugars including fructose, on brain functions and mental health." Thus, the impact fructose overconsumption could have on other organs or physiological functions has been somehow neglected. It has been reported that when consumed in low amount, the intestine metabolizes fructose into glucose with almost no fructose spill over into the bloodstream. Even if spill over may happen in the portal vein, fructose will be metabolized and transformed into fatty acids by the liver. Nevertheless, when consumed in excess, fructose spills over into the bloodstream and may enter organs including the brain [39].

The fact that the brain is fully equipped to uptake and metabolize fructose supports the concept that fructose could affect the activity of brain networks. The main fructose transporter GLUT5 and the ketohexokinase (KHK, the principal fructose-metabolizing enzyme) are expressed in the brain and at the BBB [40]. Both human and animal studies have shown that the brain reacts to high fructose intake. For instance, studies from K Page showed that fructose ingestion does activate some brain regions but which are different to the one activated by a glucose load [41, 42]. Interestingly, they showed that fructose load does not decrease the hunger sensation as compared to glucose. This would suggest that fructose does not send a satiety signal to the brain as powerful as glucose does. In support of this, studies in animal models showed that intracerebral injection of fructose stimulates food intake [43, 44]. Fructose overconsumption may also alter other brain functions including cognition and mood. Studies showed that rodents fed a high-fructose diet present memory deficits or anxiety-related behaviors [45–49]. Interestingly, it seems that the adolescence may be a more sensitive period to high fructose exposition [47, 49, 50]. This is particularly puzzling since adolescents are the population eating fructose and transformed food the most. Nevertheless, in all these animal studies with high-fructose feeding, the effect of fructose diet cannot be segregated from its impact of glucose homeostasis. It is not clear yet whether fructose may directly alter neuronal network. Many more studies need to be performed to fully understand the direct effect of fructose on brain cells and the brain functions impaired by fructose overconsumption. In addition, many other questions have not been answered yet. Can fructose be used as glucose to fuel brain cells, even though its basal blood level is extremely low? Do fructose-sensing neurons or glial cells exist within the brain? These open questions must be answered rapidly in order to improve the nutritional recommendation regarding the consumption of this sugar.

6. Conclusions

Over the last 50 years or so, our vision of the impact of sugars on the brain has significantly evolved. Knowing for its fueling role to brain cells, glucose is also considered as a signaling molecule informing the brain of the whole-body energy status and availability thanks to the discoveries of specialized glucose-sensing neurons. The findings that not only neurons are able to sense changes in glucose level and the fact that glial or neuronal glucose sensors are present all over the brain show the importance of detecting glucose level for a proper control of energy homeostasis. Nowadays, the nutritional mutation we are facing raises other concerns. The brain would be somehow protected to glucose overconsumption in view of the transporter present at the blood-brain barrier, which is saturated around 2–2.5 mM. However, the impact on brain of the metabolic changes induced by such increase in sugar consumption is yet to be evaluated further. Which brain networks and brain functions are altered by increased sugar consumption? In addition, the change in the nature of the sugars we eat raises others questions as described here for fructose. Years of research are still needed to improve our understanding of the impact of sugars on the brain in order to propose optimal nutritional recommendations.

Acknowledgements

The authors are thankful to C. Bosh-Bouju and S. Layé for the invitation to write a chapter in the book they are editing.

Conflict of interest

The authors declare no conflict of interest.

Author details

Xavier Fioramonti[1*] and Luc Pénicaud[2]

1 Université de Bordeaux, INRA, Bordeaux INP, NutriNeuro, UMR 1286, Bordeaux, France

2 UMR STROMALab, Université de Toulouse, CNRS ERL5311, EFS, INP-ENVT, Inserm U1031, UPS, Toulouse, France

*Address all correspondence to: xavier.fioramonti@inra.fr

References

[1] Mergenthaler P, Lindauer U, Dienel GA, Meisel A. Sugar for the brain: The role of glucose in physiological and pathological brain function. Trends in Neurosciences. 2013;**36**:587-597. DOI: 10.1016/j.tins.2013.07.001

[2] Levin BE. Metabolic sensing neurons and the control of energy homeostasis. Physiology & Behavior. 2006;**89**:486-489. DOI: 10.1016/j.physbeh.2006.07.003

[3] Penicaud L, Leloup C, Lorsignol A, Alquier T, Guillod E. Brain glucose sensing mechanism and glucose homeostasis. Current Opinion in Clinical Nutrition and Metabolic Care. 2002;**5**:539-543

[4] Bentsen MA, Mirzadeh Z, Schwartz MW. Revisiting how the brain senses glucose-and why. Cell Metabolism. 2019;**29**:11-17. DOI: 10.1016/j.cmet.2018.11.001

[5] Thorens B, Mueckler M. Glucose transporters in the 21st Century. American Journal of Physiology-Endocrinology and Metabolism. 2010;**298**:E141-E145. DOI: 10.1152/ajpendo.00712.2009

[6] Vogt MC, Bruning JC. CNS insulin signaling in the control of energy homeostasis and glucose metabolism—From embryo to old age. Trends in Endocrinology and Metabolism. 2013;**24**:76-84. DOI: 10.1016/j.tem.2012.11.004

[7] Kullmann S, Heni M, Hallschmid M, Fritsche A, Preissl H, Haring HU. Brain insulin resistance at the crossroads of metabolic and cognitive disorders in humans. Physiological Reviews. 2016;**96**:1169-1209. DOI: 10.1152/physrev.00032.2015

[8] de la Monte SM, Tong M, Schiano I, Didsbury J. Improved brain insulin/IGF signaling and reduced neuroinflammation with T3D-959 in an experimental model of sporadic Alzheimer's disease. Journal of Alzheimer's Disease. 2017;**55**:849-864. DOI: 10.3233/JAD-160656

[9] Garcia-Caceres C, Balland E, Prevot V, Luquet S, Woods SC, Koch M, et al. Role of astrocytes, microglia, and tanycytes in brain control of systemic metabolism. Nature Neuroscience. 2019;**22**:7-14. DOI: 10.1038/s41593-018-0286-y

[10] Pellerin L, Magistretti PJ. Sweet sixteen for ANLS. Journal of Cerebral Blood Flow & Metabolism. 2012;**32**:1152-1166. DOI: 10.1038/jcbfm.2011.149

[11] Oomura Y, Kimura K, Ooyama H, Maeo T, Iki M, Kuniyoshi N. Reciprocal activities of the ventromedial and lateral hypothalamic area of cats. Science. 1964;**143**:484-485

[12] Anand BK, Chhina GS, Sharma KN, Dua S, Singh B. Activity of single neurons in the hypothalamic feeding centers: Effect of glucose. American Journal of Physiology-Legacy Content. 1964;**207**:1146-1154

[13] Oomura Y, Ooyama H, Sugimori M, Nakamura T, Yamada Y. Glucose inhibition of the glucose-sensitive neurone in the rat lateral hypothalamus. Nature. 1974;**247**:284-286

[14] de Vries MG, Arseneau LM, Lawson ME, Beverly JL. Extracellular glucose in rat ventromedial hypothalamus during acute and recurrent hypoglycemia. Diabetes. 2003;**52**:2767-2773

[15] Dunn-Meynell AA, Sanders NM, Compton D, Becker TC, Eiki J, Zhang BB, et al. Relationship among brain and blood glucose levels and spontaneous and glucoprivic feeding. Journal of

Neuroscience. 2009;**29**:7015-7022. DOI: 10.1523/JNEUROSCI.0334-09.2009

[16] Langlet F, Levin BE, Luquet S, Mazzone M, Messina A, Dunn-Meynell AA, et al. Tanycytic VEGF-A boosts blood-hypothalamus barrier plasticity and access of metabolic signals to the arcuate nucleus in response to fasting. Cell Metabolism. 2013;**17**:607-617. DOI: 10.1016/j.cmet.2013.03.004

[17] McNay EC, Gold PE. Extracellular glucose concentrations in the rat hippocampus measured by zero-net-flux: Effects of microdialysis flow rate, strain, and age. Journal of Neurochemistry. 1999;**72**:785-790

[18] McNay EC, McCarty RC, Gold PE. Fluctuations in brain glucose concentration during behavioral testing: Dissociations between brain areas and between brain and blood. Neurobiology of Learning and Memory. 2001;**75**:325-337

[19] Routh VH. Glucose-sensing neurons: Are they physiologically relevant? Physiology & Behavior. 2002;**76**:403-413. DOI: S0031938402007618 [pii]

[20] Fioramonti X, Chretien C, Leloup C, Penicaud L. Recent advances in the cellular and molecular mechanisms of hypothalamic neuronal glucose detection. Frontiers in Physiology. 2017;**8**:875. DOI: 10.3389/fphys.2017.00875

[21] Routh VH, Hao L, Santiago AM, Sheng Z, Zhou C. Hypothalamic glucose sensing: Making ends meet. Frontiers in Systems Neuroscience. 2014;**8**:236. DOI: 10.3389/fnsys.2014.00236

[22] Wang R, Liu X, Hentges ST, Dunn-Meynell AA, Levin BE, Wang W, et al. The regulation of glucose-excited neurons in the hypothalamic arcuate nucleus by glucose and feeding-relevant peptides. Diabetes. 2004;**53**:1959-1965

[23] Fioramonti X, Lorsignol A, Taupignon A, Penicaud L. A new ATP-sensitive K+ channel-independent mechanism is involved in glucose-excited neurons of mouse arcuate nucleus. Diabetes. 2004;**53**:2767-2775. DOI: 53/11/2767 [pii]

[24] Penicaud L, Leloup C, Fioramonti X, Lorsignol A, Benani A. Brain glucose sensing: A subtle mechanism. Current Opinion in Clinical Nutrition and Metabolic Care. 2006;**9**:458-462

[25] Chretien C, Fenech C, Lienard F, Grall S, Chevalier C, Chaudy S, et al. Transient receptor potential canonical 3 (TRPC3) channels are required for hypothalamic glucose detection and energy homeostasis. Diabetes. 2017;**66**:314-324. DOI: 10.2337/db16-1114

[26] Ciofi P. The arcuate nucleus as a circumventricular organ in the mouse. Neuroscience Letters. 2011;**487**:187-190. DOI: 10.1016/j.neulet.2010.10.019

[27] Song Z, Levin BE, McArdle JJ, Bakhos N, Routh VH. Convergence of pre- and postsynaptic influences on glucosensing neurons in the ventromedial hypothalamic nucleus. Diabetes. 2001;**50**:2673-2681

[28] Arluison M, Quignon M, Nguyen P, Thorens B, Leloup C, Penicaud L. Distribution and anatomical localization of the glucose transporter 2 (GLUT2) in the adult rat brain—An immunohistochemical study. Journal of Chemical Neuroanatomy. 2004;**28**:117-136

[29] Arluison M, Quignon M, Thorens B, Leloup C, Penicaud L. Immunocytochemical localization of the glucose transporter 2 (GLUT2) in the adult rat brain. II. Electron microscopic study. Journal of Chemical Neuroanatomy. 2004;**28**:137-146

[30] Leloup C, Arluison M, Lepetit N, Cartier N, Marfaing-Jallat P, Ferre P,

et al. Glucose transporter 2 (GLUT 2): Expression in specific brain nuclei. Brain Research. 1994;**638**:221-226

[31] Guillod-Maximin E, Lorsignol A, Alquier T, Penicaud L. Acute intracarotid glucose injection towards the brain induces specific c-fos activation in hypothalamic nuclei: Involvement of astrocytes in cerebral glucose-sensing in rats. Journal of Neuroendocrinology. 2004;**16**:464-471. DOI: 10.1111/j.1365-2826.2004.01185.x

[32] Frayling C, Britton R, Dale N. ATP-mediated glucosensing by hypothalamic tanycytes. The Journal of Physiology. 2011;**589**:2275-2286. DOI: 10.1113/jphysiol.2010.202051

[33] Orellana JA, Saez PJ, Cortes-Campos C, Elizondo RJ, Shoji KF, Contreras-Duarte S, et al. Glucose increases intracellular free Ca(2+) in tanycytes via ATP released through connexin 43 hemichannels. Glia. 2012;**60**:53-68. DOI: 10.1002/glia.21246

[34] Bouyakdan K, Martin H, Lienard F, Budry L, Taib B, Rodaros D, et al. The gliotransmitter ACBP controls feeding and energy homeostasis via the melanocortin system. Journal of Clinical Investigation. 2019;**130**:2417-2430. DOI: 10.1172/JCI123454

[35] Lanfray D, Arthaud S, Ouellet J, Compere V, Do Rego JL, Leprince J, et al. Gliotransmission and brain glucose sensing: Critical role of endozepines. Diabetes. 2013;**62**:801-810. DOI: 10.2337/db11-0785

[36] Yang XJ, Kow LM, Funabashi T, Mobbs CV. Hypothalamic glucose sensor: Similarities to and differences from pancreatic beta-cell mechanisms. Diabetes. 1999;**48**:1763-1772

[37] Li Q, Cheng Z, Zhou L, Darmanis S, Neff NF, Okamoto J, et al. Developmental heterogeneity of microglia and brain myeloid cells revealed by deep single-cell RNA sequencing. Neuron. 2019;**101**:207-223.e10. DOI: 10.1016/j.neuron.2018.12.006

[38] Tappy L. Fructose metabolism and noncommunicable diseases: Recent findings and new research perspectives. Current Opinion in Clinical Nutrition and Metabolic Care. 2018;**21**:214-222. DOI: 10.1097/MCO.0000000000000460

[39] Jang C, Hui S, Lu W, Cowan AJ, Morscher RJ, Lee G, et al. The small intestine converts dietary fructose into glucose and organic acids. Cell Metabolism. 2018;**27**:351-361.e3. DOI: 10.1016/j.cmet.2017.12.016

[40] Oppelt SA, Zhang W, Tolan DR. Specific regions of the brain are capable of fructose metabolism. Brain Research. 2017;**1657**:312-322. DOI: 10.1016/j.brainres.2016.12.022

[41] Page KA, Chan O, Arora J, Belfort-Deaguiar R, Dzuira J, Roehmholdt B, et al. Effects of fructose vs glucose on regional cerebral blood flow in brain regions involved with appetite and reward pathways. JAMA. 2013;**309**:63-70. DOI: 10.1001/jama.2012.116975

[42] Luo S, Monterosso JR, Sarpelleh K, Page KA. Differential effects of fructose versus glucose on brain and appetitive responses to food cues and decisions for food rewards. Proceedings of the National Academy of Sciences. 2015;**112**:6509-6514. DOI: 10.1073/pnas.1503358112

[43] Miller CC, Martin RJ, Whitney ML, Edwards GL. Intracerebroventricular injection of fructose stimulates feeding in rats. Nutritional Neuroscience. 2002;**5**:359-362. DOI: 10.1080/1028415021000033839

[44] Cha SH, Wolfgang M, Tokutake Y, Chohnan S, Lane MD. Differential effects of central fructose and glucose on hypothalamic malonyl-CoA and

food intake. Proceedings of the National Academy of Sciences. 2008;**105**: 16871-16875. DOI: 10.1073/pnas.0809255105

[45] Lowette K, Roosen L, Tack J, Vanden Berghe P. Effects of high-fructose diets on central appetite signaling and cognitive function. Frontiers in Nutrition. 2015;**2**:5. DOI: 10.3389/fnut.2015.00005

[46] Wu HW, Ren LF, Zhou X, Han DW. A high-fructose diet induces hippocampal insulin resistance and exacerbates memory deficits in male Sprague-Dawley rats. Nutritional Neuroscience. 2015;**18**:323-328. DOI: 10.1179/1476830514Y.0000000133

[47] Harrell CS, Burgado J, Kelly SD, Johnson ZP, Neigh GN. High-fructose diet during periadolescent development increases depressive-like behavior and remodels the hypothalamic transcriptome in male rats. Psychoneuroendocrinology. 2015;**62**:252-264. DOI: 10.1016/j.psyneuen.2015.08.025

[48] Hsu TM, Konanur VR, Taing L, Usui R, Kayser BD, Goran MI, et al. Effects of sucrose and high fructose corn syrup consumption on spatial memory function and hippocampal neuroinflammation in adolescent rats. Hippocampus. 2015;**25**:227-239. DOI: 10.1002/hipo.22368

[49] Reddy BR, Maitra S, Jhelum P, Kumar KP, Bagul PK, Kaur G, et al. Sirtuin 1 and 7 mediate resveratrol-induced recovery from hyper-anxiety in high-fructose-fed prediabetic rats. Journal of Biosciences. 2016;**41**:407-417

[50] Zemdegs J, Quesseveur G, Jarriault D, Penicaud L, Fioramonti X, Guiard BP. High-fat diet-induced metabolic disorders impairs 5-HT function and anxiety-like behavior in mice. British Journal of Pharmacology. 2016;**173**:2095-2110. DOI: 10.1111/bph.13343

Section 4

Diet and Autophagy in the Brain

Chapter 4

Dietary Impact on Neuronal Autophagy Control and Brain Health

Claudia Ntsapi, Andre du Toit and Ben Loos

Abstract

Autophagy is the major intracellular system which is critical for the removal of harmful protein aggregates and malfunctioning organelles. Dysfunctional autophagy is associated with a multitude of human diseases, such as protein aggregation in Alzheimer's disease and non-successful aging. Major interest exists in the dietary manipulation of the autophagy pathway activity, so as to tune the cell's protein degradation capabilities and to prevent cell death onset. It has recently become clear that the machinery required to degrade protein cargo has a distinct activity level which can be altered through specific dietary modulation. Moreover, this activity may differ from that of the proteinaceous cargo. Overall, brain health and successful aging are characterized by limited protein aggregation, with a distinct molecular signature of maintained autophagy function. However, it is largely unclear how to control autophagy through dietary interventions with a precision that would allow to maintain minimal levels of toxic proteins, preserving neuronal cell viability and proteostasis. In this chapter, we carefully dissect the relationship between autophagy-modulating drugs, including caloric restriction mimetics and their impact on neuronal autophagy, in the context of preserving brain health.

Keywords: autophagic flux, caloric restriction, proteotoxicity, Alzheimer's disease, neurodegeneration, autophagosome, lysosome

1. Introduction

At the beginning of the twentieth century, life expectancy at birth was about 45 years. Today, this figure has markedly increased to nearly 77 years [1]. Recent estimates [1] predict that in the next four decades, the world's proportion of people aged 65 years and older will account for nearly 22% of the total population—from the present 800 million to 2 billion people. Although this increase in life expectancy is reflective of the healthcare achievements [2], the socioeconomic costs associated with a higher chronic disease burden have necessitated the development of robust prevention and management strategies that are both safe and immediately executable.

2. The role of protein aggregation in Alzheimer's disease

Alzheimer's disease (AD) is a debilitating neurodegenerative disease, affecting 40 million people worldwide [3]. The prevalence of AD is strongly correlated with age, imposing a greater socioeconomic burden as life expectancy continues to increase. Clinically, AD is associated with the progressive loss of essential cognitive functions and progressive hippocampal and cortical brain atrophy [4]. Current AD treatment Food and Drug Administration (FDA)-approved drugs include N-methyl-D-aspartic acid (NMDA) receptor antagonist memantine and cholinesterase inhibitors donepezil, galantamine, and rivastigmine [5]. These drugs augment cholinergic neurotransmission or attenuate excitotoxic neuronal injury. However, they only provide palliative benefits at best, with limited impact on the underlying disease mechanisms. Therefore, there is an urgent need for interventions that not only impact the aging process in favor of sustained brain health but also promote successful brain aging in the context of neurodegenerative diseases. AD is pathologically defined by the widespread brain distribution of amyloid-beta peptide (Aβ) plaques, neurofibrillary tangle (NFT) formation, as well as synaptic and neuronal loss [6]. Despite growing understanding of the disease, it remains unclear how these pathological features relate to the specific disease processes. The amyloid cascade hypothesis continues to serve as the predominant model of AD pathology. This hypothesis suggests the overproduction of Aβ, particularly an increase in Aβ [42] relative to Aβ [40], as the causal trigger in the disease process [7]. Aβ is derived from the amyloidogenic cleavage of the amyloid precursor protein (APP), protein cleaved by two endoproteases: the beta-site APP-cleaving enzyme 1 (BACE1/β-secretase) and γ-secretase enzyme. Briefly, APP is cleaved by BACE1, releasing sAPPβ and leaving the membrane-bound C99 carboxy-terminal fragment that is subsequently processed by γ-secretase to generate Aβ, a nontoxic P3 peptide, and the APP intracellular domain (AICD) [7]. γ-Secretase cleavage results in a C-terminal heterogeneity of the resulting Aβ peptide population. Hence, Aβ peptides of different lengths exist, with Aβ40 being the most abundant (~80–90%), followed by the more hydrophobic and fibrillogenic Aβ42 (~5–10%) form which is the principal peptide aggregated in the AD brain [8].

Similar to AD, protein aggregation is also a hallmark of neuronal cell death onset in Parkinson's disease (PD). PD is pathologically defined by the formation of intraneuronal inclusions consisting of aggregated α-synuclein (α-syn) and the presence of Lewy neurites and Lewy bodies (LBs) [9]. This neuropathology is associated with impaired functioning of intracellular protein degradation mechanisms [10]. Thus, strategies to either degrade or prevent the initial accumulation of Aβ oligomers and α-syn may be promising in the treatment or prevention of AD and PD, respectively.

3. Protein quality surveillance machinery

The postmitotic nature of neuronal cells makes them highly susceptible to the accumulation of protein aggregates. Hence, the maintenance of protein homeostasis is critical to maintain neuronal function, particularly with age. Although the etiology and molecular mechanisms underlying the pathological changes in AD are not fully understood, studies suggest that localized deficits in the autophagy pathway are likely to precede the formation of Aβ plaques or NFTs [11]. Autophagy is a highly conserved catabolic process that is critical for the systemic removal of long-lived proteins, protein aggregates, and dysfunctional organelles and serves as a major regulator of longevity in various species [12]. This process is triggered by various stressors, e.g., low nutrient levels, and proteotoxicity [13]. Proteotoxicity is by the of functional conformation as mature proteins misfold due to normal aging, posttranslational modifications, or inherent mutations [14]. In the absence of intracellular corrective mechanisms, this proteotoxicity can lead to uncontrolled protein aggregation, impair the cells' ability to maintain protein homeostasis, and promote cell death onset [14]. Depending on the cargo sequestered, and the mechanism

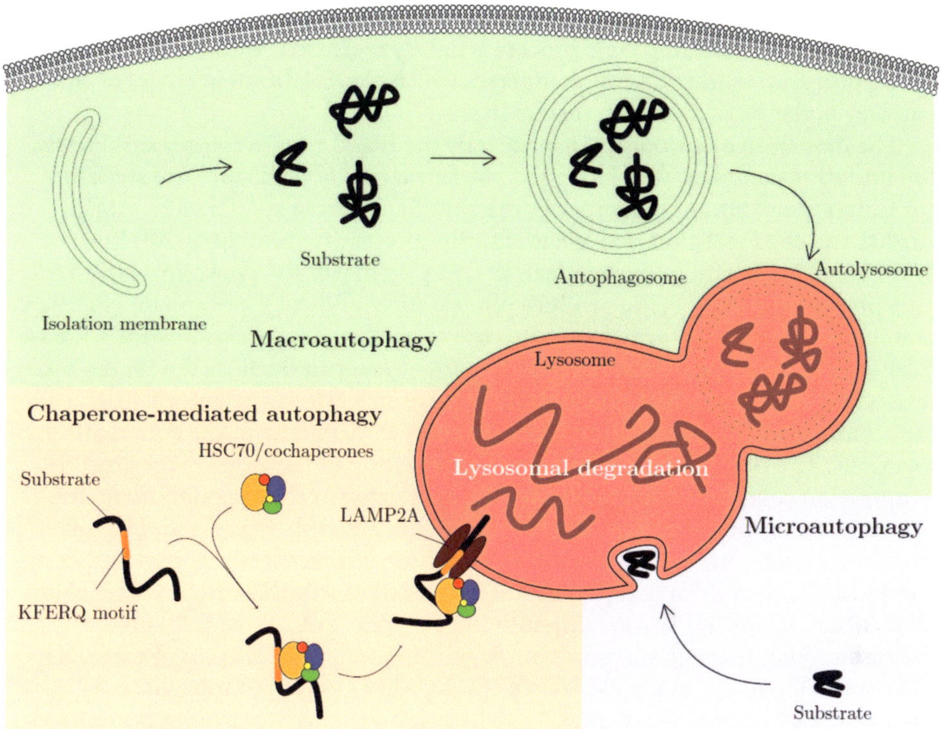

Figure 1.
Schematic model of the three main types of autophagy described in mammalian cells.

through which cargo is delivered to the lysosome, autophagy encompasses at least three subtypes: microautophagy, chaperone-mediated autophagy (CMA), and macroautophagy (**Figure 1**).

In microautophagy, lysosomal membrane invaginations mediate the internalization of cytosolic cargo into small vesicles that detach into the lumen for degradation [15]. CMA refers to a selective form of autophagy, whereby cytosolic proteins containing a CMA targeting motif—an amino-acid sequence biochemically similar to KFERQ—are bound by heat shock-cognate chaperone of 70 kDa (HSC70). HSC70 targets these proteins to the lysosomal membrane, where after binding to the cytosolic tail of lysosome-associated membrane protein type-2A (LAMP2A), proteins are unfolded and translocated across the lysosomal membrane aided by the lysosome-resident form of HSC70 (lys-hsc70) for degradation by the luminal proteases [16]. Of the three pathways, macroautophagy (hereafter referred to as autophagy) is the most extensively characterized and most relevant to AD. Therefore, this review will focus on the role of macroautophagy as the key mechanism which may be exploited to promote brain health and successful brain aging.

4. The tight orchestration of autophagy

Autophagy serves as the cell's principal quality control system which mediates the degradation of entire cytoplasmic materials through a series of stages characterized by the *de novo* formation of double-membraned vesicles, termed autophagosomes, which sequester cytoplasmic cargo and fuse with lysosomes to form autolysosomes. This process culminates in cargo degradation and subsequent recycling of the resulting macromolecules. To date, more than 30 highly conserved autophagy-related (ATG) genes have been implicated in the core autophagy machinery [17]. The autophagic process is tightly regulated, with distinct sets of Atg proteins forming diverse complexes which control different stages of this pathway under basal and stressful conditions.

The induction of autophagy is primarily mediated by two complexes. Firstly, the initiation complex, which triggers the formation of a phagophore structure (or isolation membrane), comprises the Unc-51-like kinase-1 (ULK1), Atg13, Atg101 and the focal adhesion kinase family-interacting protein of 200 kDa (FIP200) [17]. Secondly, the nucleation complex drives the phosphorylation of phosphatidylinositol (PI) to produce phosphatidylinositol 3-phosphate (PI3P), a membrane-bound lipid which requires the class III phosphatidylinositol 3-kinase (C3PI3K) vacuolar protein sorting 34 (Vps34) to recruit Beclin1, Vps15, Atg14L, or Ambra1 in the region of phagophore formation, termed the omegasome [17]. Autophagosome formation is mediated by two ubiquitin-like conjugation reactions. The first reaction results in the formation of the Atg12-Atg5-Atg16L1 conjugation complex which facilitates the expansion of the phagophore membrane. In the second reaction, Atg12-Atg5 associates with Atg16L1 and localizes to the outer membrane of the pre-autophagosomal structures, in turn catalyzing the recruitment and conjugation of microtubule-associated protein 1 light chain 3 (MAP1LC3/Atg8/LC3) with a membrane phospholipid, phosphatidylethanolamine (PE), through the action of Atg4, Atg7, and Atg3 [18]. Atg4 catalyzes the conversion of the cytosolic form of LC3 (LC3-I) to the autophagosome membrane-associated form (LC3-II), which serves as an indicator of autophagosome pool size at a given time [18]. Mature autophagosomes ultimately fuse with lysosomes to form autolysosomes, in which sequestered cargo is degraded and released back into the cytosol for reuse [18]. Autophagic flux, the rate of protein degradation through the autophagy pathway [19, 20], provides an accurate measure of this dynamic process.

5. Key signaling pathways in the regulation of autophagy during nutrient stress

The mammalian target of rapamycin complex 1 (mTORC1) is a component of mTOR, the master regulator of cellular metabolism in response to environmental cues. mTORC1 integrates various signaling networks to promote protein synthesis by suppressing catabolic processes under nutrient-rich conditions [21]. In addition to the class I phosphatidylinositol-3-kinase (PI3K) and the Akt signaling pathway, the tuberous sclerosis (TSC) tumor suppressor complex (TSC1/TSC2) is an important upstream regulator of mTORC1, with loss-of-function mutations in either complex leading to the constitutive activation of mTORC1 [22]. Under conditions of nutrient excess, growth factors such as insulin-like growth factor 1 (insulin/IGF1) activate their cognate receptors, subsequently activating the PI3K/Akt pathway [23]. Activated Akt inhibits TSC1/TSC2, resulting in the activation of mTORC1 [23]. Subsequently, mTORC1 suppresses autophagy activity by phosphorylating (i) components of the ULK1 complex; (ii) Atg14L or Beclin1 regulator (Ambra1); (iii) the Beclin1-binding protein, UV radiation resistance-associated gene (UVRAG); or (iv) the transcription factor EB (TFEB), a key regulator of lysosomal and autophagy gene expression [24]. Therefore, mTORC1 can inhibit autophagy by targeting different components of the core autophagy machinery (**Figure 2**).

Under conditions of nutrient stress, mTORC1 activity is suppressed, resulting in the activation of the ULK1 complex [24]. Cellular energetic sensor, AMP-activated protein kinase (AMPK), positively regulates autophagy to maintain energy

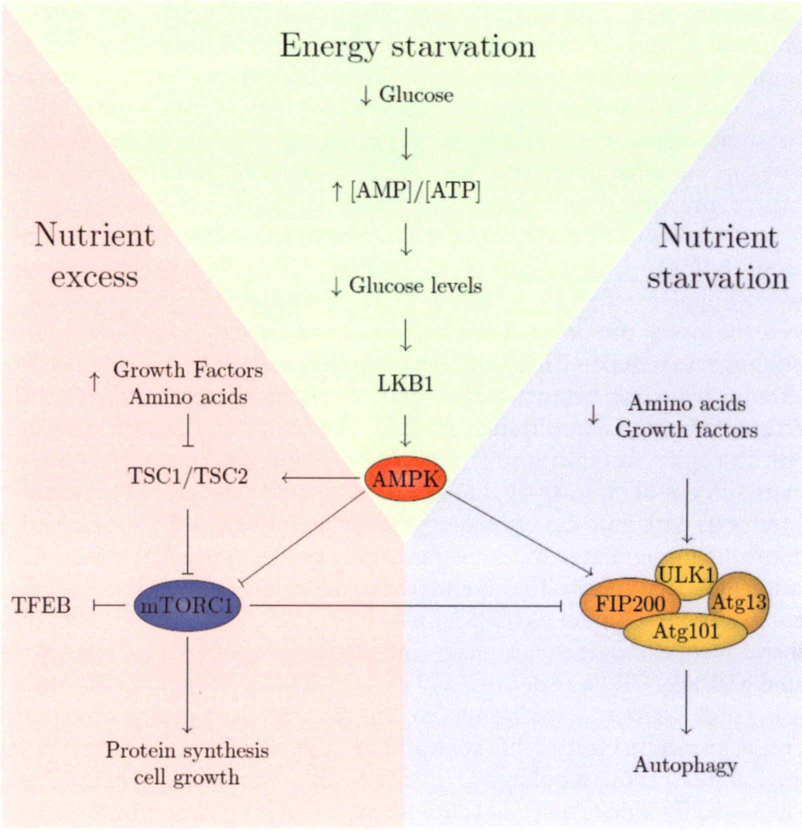

Figure 2.
Regulation of autophagy by cellular nutrient status.

homeostasis under energy depleted conditions. Briefly, AMPK phosphorylates TSC2- and mTORC1-binding partner regulatory-associated protein (Raptor) [25], thereby suppressing mTORC1 activity. Additionally, AMPK can bind and phosphorylate ULK1, freeing this complex to initiate autophagy under both nutrient and ATP deplete conditions [26]. Thus, initiation of autophagy can be jointly regulated by mTORC1 and AMPK, to increase the cell's capacity to adapt to metabolic perturbations.

6. Decreased autophagy with age

Consistent with the transcriptional downregulation of autophagy during healthy aging in the human brain [27], the impairment of autophagy has been found to decrease life span in various model systems [28]. Screening for chronological aging factors, Matecic et al. [29] published one of the earliest findings implicating impaired autophagy activity in the shortened life span of *S. cerevisiae* mutants. Most compelling findings came from Atg5 [30] or Atg7 [31] knockout mice which revealed that impaired autophagic function led to early postnatal death, the accumulation of intracellular inclusion bodies, and neurodegeneration. Since insufficient/impaired autophagy contributes to aging, it is conceivable that increasing the activity of this process could influence aging, in favor of life span extension. Indeed, it is becoming increasingly clear that modulation strategies that enhance autophagy activity attenuate proteotoxicity, while defects in this pathway have been implicated in increased risk for cell death onset with age [28]. Autophagy dysfunction has been extensively documented in AD progression, where the accumulation of incompletely degraded cytoplasmic within autophagic vacuoles (AVs) has been shown to be a pathological hallmark of insufficient autophagic induction in AD [32]. This process is further exacerbated by the presence of APP and its processing enzymes within the AVs [33], indicating that autophagy may regulate both Aβ generation and clearance. Indeed, insufficient expression of autophagy core protein Beclin1 has been shown to increase the expression levels of APP, Aβ, and the C-terminal fragment (CTF) in cultured neurons, in early AD patients, and mouse models of AD, while Beclin1 overexpression had the opposite effect [34]. Therefore, the modulation of autophagy may ameliorate the loss of proteostasis in AD. Indeed, rapamycin, an mTORC1 inhibitor, has been shown to reduce Aβ load and tau pathology and improve cognitive function [35], with this reduction being most pronounced when rapamycin was administered prior to the widespread deposition of Aβ [36]. Therefore, the identification of novel treatment strategies, or repurposing of readily available autophagy-inducing drugs to promote successful brain aging, has attracted considerable attention. Additionally, drugs/strategies with dual-functional capabilities in both the inhibition of Aβ production and upregulation of its clearance may prove especially beneficial in the attenuation of Aβ pathology. To this end, the use of calorie restriction (CR) dietary interventions and CR mimetics (CRMs) may offer a relatively simple, safe, and inexpensive avenue to induce autophagy and offset the decline of autophagy activity associated with age. CR, here defined as a reduction in caloric/energetic intake without causing malnutrition, remains not only the most robust and reproducible dietary intervention known to increase life span and delay aging but is also a most potent physiological inducer of autophagy [37]. In fact, short-term fasting in mice has been shown to markedly induce neuronal autophagy, translating in neuroprotection [38].

7. CR effects on aging and neurodegeneration

7.1 CR regimes

Intermittent fasting (IF) is the most studied CR regime in humans. IF involves alternating between periods of *ad libitum* (AL) caloric intake and partial or complete CR in which food intake is restricted for prolonged time periods [39]. The majority of IF animal studies have involved either alternating IF (AIF) or time-restricted intermittent fasting (TRIF), with both resulting in neuroprotection, as evidenced by the enhancement of neuronal plasticity, increased levels of brain-derived neurotrophic factor (BDNF), and increased resistance to metabolic stress [40]. Goodrick and colleagues revealed that rats maintained on a lifelong AIF regime lived nearly twice as long as rats fed AL [41]. More recently, CR regimes have also been shown to attenuate Aβ neuropathology in the brains of AD mouse models [42]. In agreement, AD mice maintained for 1 year on either AIF or a 40% CR diet beginning from 5 months of age were not found to exhibit the cognitive impairments observed in AL fed AD mice [43]. However, the beneficial effects of CR on aging and maximal life span in humans remain unclear given the ethical controversies associated with long-term survival studies in normal-weight humans, the lack of validated biomarkers of aging, and the limited compliance to prolonged CR regimes [44]. Notably, gender-based differences have been reported in response to CR regimes [45]. For example, work by Martin et al. [46] revealed that while male and female rats maintained on a CR regime for 6 months had similar levels of circulating triglycerides and energy-regulating hormones (insulin, leptin, adiponectin, and ghrelin), the changes were quantitatively greater in males.

The most compelling support for the beneficial effects of CR on longevity stems from epidemiological studies of the older Okinawan population, which is the longest lived population to date [47]. The longevity and apparent rarity of progressive neurodegenerative diseases amongst? this population are associated with strict adherence to their traditional Okinawan diet, consisting of soybean-based foods, unrefined carbohydrates, and moderate protein intake with emphasis on root vegetables (sweet potatoes), fish, and lean meats [48]. However, given the paucity of long-term CR studies in humans, there is insufficient data to determine the optimal CR regimen and the degree of CR needed to achieve sustained brain health.

7.2 CR and brain health

During the aging process, neuronal cells are exposed to increased oxidative and metabolic stress associated with numerous cellular modifications [49]. These modifications are aggravated in neurodegenerative diseases, where neuronal injury is most pronounced in the hippocampus and cortex region. Strong evidence from animal studies suggests that CR promotes enhanced synaptic plasticity, resulting in increased brain resistance to metabolic stressors, and delays brain aging [50]. Studies suggest that long-term CR, from 3 to 11 months of age, had a survival-promoting effect on newly formed glial cells in the hippocampus region of 2-, 18-, and 24-month-old mice [51]. In AD mouse models maintained on a 6–14 week CR regime, a significant reduction in Aβ and astrocytic activation was observed [52]. Hence, exploitation of the mechanisms through which CR augments brain health may aid in the development of lifestyle-based therapeutics in the treatment of AD and other neurodegenerative diseases. Although the exact mechanisms through which CR promotes health and life span are not fully understood, nutrient signaling pathways have been implicated (**Figure 3**). Of considerable importance to the CR-induced effects on brain aging is the induction of autophagy following the activation of metabolic energy sensors AMPK and sirtuin-1 (SIRT1) or the inhibition of the insulin/IGF1 pathway and mTORC1 signaling [53].

7.3 SIRT1

SIRT1 is a nicotine amide NAD^+-dependent histone deacetylase, which exhibits increased expression following CR in many tissues, including the brain [54]. Importantly, SIRT1 overexpression has also been shown to promote autophagy by activating essential Atg proteins [55]. SIRT1 can further stimulate autophagy by deacetylating and activating the Forkhead box (FOXO) family of transcription factors which act as key regulators of longevity under CR conditions [56]. SIRT1 may further promote longevity through FOXO-dependent induction of stress response genes [56].

7.4 AMPK

AMPK is activated in response to low energy levels, e.g., under CR conditions [57], suggesting that AMPK may play a role in CR-induced longevity. Indeed, increased AMPK activity has been found to extend life span in *C. elegans* and *Drosophila* model systems, while its inhibition shortened life span [58]. The mechanism underlying AMPK-induced life span extension under CR is thought to involve the direct phosphorylation of peroxisome proliferator-activated receptor G coactivator-1α (PGC-1α), a key regulator of mitochondrial metabolism and biogenesis, and FOXO transcription factors, thereby targeting these components for SIRT1-mediated activation [59]. Importantly, AMPK stimulates autophagy through the direct phosphorylation of ULK1, or the activation of TSC1/TSC2, which in turn inhibits mTORC1 [25], thereby allowing autophagy induction.

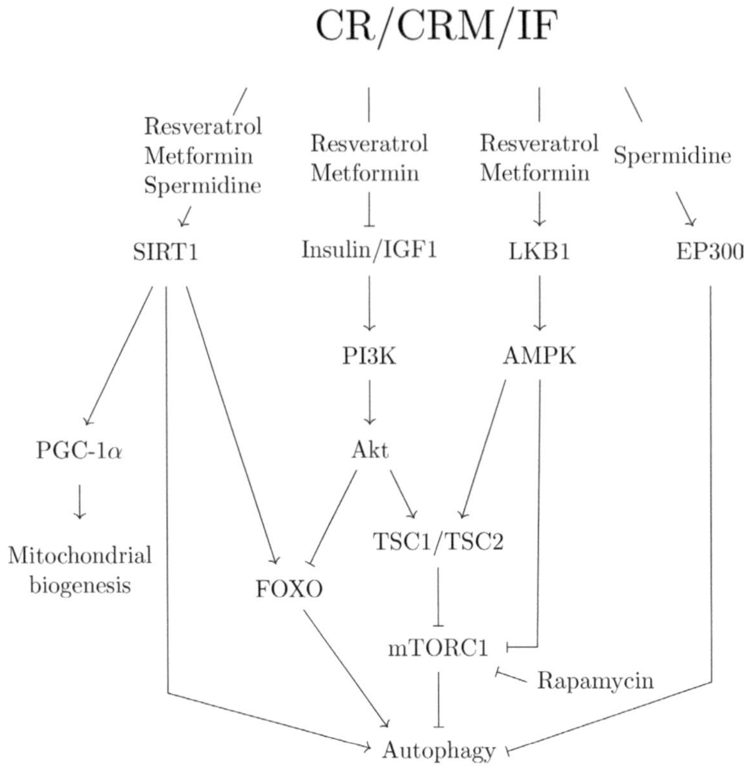

Figure 3.
The targeting of nutrient-triggered pathways by selective calorie restriction mimetics in longevity and the promotion of brain health. CR, calorie restriction; CRM, caloric restriction mimetic; IF, intermittent fasting; SIRT1, sirtuin-1; mTORC1, mammalian target of rapamycin complex 1; AMPK, AMP-dependent protein kinase; PGC-1α, peroxisome proliferator-activated receptor gamma coactivator 1-α; insulin/IGF-1, insulin/insulin-like growth factor-1; PI3K, phosphoinositide 3-kinase; FOXO, Forkhead box O; EP300, E1A-binding protein p300.

7.5 Insulin/IGF1 signaling

Inhibition of insulin/IGF1 signaling following CR or growth factor removal has been reported to increase life span, delay the onset of age-related diseases, and increase oxidative stress resistance in various species, including humans [60]. CR-induced downregulation of the insulin/IGF1 pathway in turn induces the activation of SIRT1, resulting in the activation of FOXO transcription factors [61].

7.6 mTORC1 signaling

mTORC1 is activated by growth factors, amino acids, or increased glucose levels, and is thought to control life span through various mechanisms, including the regulation of autophagy [62]. Indeed, autophagy has been shown to be essential for life span expansion in mTOR knockout yeast [63] and *C. elegans* model systems in which impaired autophagic function has been shown to abolish the life span extension induced by mTOR inhibition under CR conditions [28]. The convergence of CR-induced signaling pathways on autophagy supports the assertion that this process is intricately involved in aging. Therefore, the precision control of brain autophagy activity could mediate sustained brain health with age.

8. Antiaging pharmacological CR mimetics

Given the challenge to adhere to prolonged CR regimes, as well as selective side effects, such as decreased body temperature [64] and slowed wound healing [65], compounds that elicit similar beneficial effects on aging, health, and life span as CR could be a more practical alternative. This area of research has sparked considerable interest in the use CRM drugs, or CRM supplements as adjuvant therapy to delay the aging process, particularly during mid- to late life. Currently, the most widely studied CRM candidates are resveratrol, rapamycin, 2-deoxy-D-glucose (2DG), metformin, and spermidine (**Figure 3**).

8.1 Resveratrol

Resveratrol is a polyphenol compound isolated from the skins of red grapes, with red wine (5 mg/L on average) being the principal source of this compound [66]. Daily consumption of grape and blueberry polyphenols has also gained interest as CRMs for the prevention and treatment of neurodegenerative diseases. For example, studies indicate that the combined dietary supplementation of grape and blueberry polyphenols may have beneficial effects on age-related cognitive decline, improving episodic memory impairment in elderly subjects [67] and preventing the onset of learning and cognitive deficits in aged mice [68]. However, resveratrol has been found to be the most potent polyphenol compound and is to date the most thoroughly studied CRM, first identified and implicated in life span extension in a yeast model system [69]. Work by Baur et al. [70] revealed that resveratrol significantly increased survival in middle-aged mice on a high-calorie diet compared to that of mice on a standard diet by nearly 31%. In addition, resveratrol increased insulin sensitivity, reduced IGF1 levels, activated AMPK/PGC-1α signaling, and improved motor function [70]. Similar benefits have been reported in response to resveratrol supplementation in nonhuman primate models fed a high-fat diet [71, 72]. In the latter study, resveratrol improved adipose insulin levels and reduced the inflammatory response caused by the high-fat diet [72], while the former study revealed that resveratrol prevented diet-induced arterial wall inflammation [71].

Naturally sourced resveratrol is poorly absorbed in humans [73]. Hence, high-purity resveratrol-mimetic drugs, such as ResVida™, have been developed to ensure its sustained release [74]. In a recent study, 30-day resveratrol supplementation (150 mg/day ResVida™) in humans led to a decrease in circulating glucose levels, inflammatory markers, triglycerides, and systolic blood pressure [74]. In contrast, others have reported no significant changes in the above parameters in obese men following resveratrol supplementation [75]. Longevinex® is another commercially available resveratrol supplement shown to induce SIRT1 and PGC-1α and increase mitochondrial biogenesis in the brain [76]. Prolonged Longevinex® supplementation has been shown to result in increased levels of LC3-II, Beclin1, and FOXO transcription factors. Therefore, it appears conceivable that prolonged Longevinex® may influence brain health, in part, by inducing neuronal autophagy. Work by Vingtdeux et al. [77] has also revealed that resveratrol can decrease extracellular Aβ accumulation by inducing autophagy through the activation of AMPK. Long-term resveratrol treatment is well tolerated in humans [78], with significantly reduced Aβ levels and improved memory retention observed in AD mouse models [79], making this compound a promising CRM candidate for the treatment of AD.

8.2 Rapamycin

The suppression of mTORC1 activity is associated with a significant improvement in both health and life span in various organisms, while increased activity is associated with old age in humans [80]. Hence, the use of mTORC1 inhibitor rapamycin may have potential applications as a CRM. Currently, rapamycin is clinically used as an immunosuppressant to prevent the rejection of kidney transplants in patients [66]. In AD mouse models, rapamycin treatment has been shown to improve cognitive ability and reduce Aβ and tau pathology, with these observations being linked to increased autophagic induction [81]. However, it has been reported that prolonged rapamycin treatment in rodents leads to the development of hyperlipidemia, glucose intolerance, and high levels of free fatty acids in skeletal muscle [82]. In contrast, lifelong intermittent administration of rapamycin for 2 weeks/month was found to extend life span in mice [81], suggesting that intermittent rapamycin administration may be more beneficial. In a separate study, adult mice maintained on lifelong rapamycin treatment, starting at 2 months of age, performed significantly better on a task measuring spatial learning and memory compared to age-matched mice on the control diet [83]. However, rapamycin did not improve cognition in adult mice with pre-existing age-dependent cognitive deficits [83], suggesting that rapamycin may have better cognitive outcomes prior to the onset of cognitive deficits.

Rapamycin is unstable in water; thus, different oral preparations such as nanoparticles [84] have been formulated to increase its bioavailability. Rapatar, a rapamycin formulation based on Pluronic block copolymers as nanocarriers, has been shown to have significantly higher bioavailability after oral administration [85]. Rapatar has been shown to increase life span and delay carcinogenesis during lifelong treatment administered at intermittently low doses (0.5 mg/kg) in tumor-prone mice [86]. The advantage of rapamycin is its FDA-approved status for various clinical applications in humans; however, the relevance for longevity in humans has yet to be established given its immunosuppressive effects.

8.3 Metformin

Metformin is a first-line drug approved for the treatment of diabetes [87], which also targets the insulin/IGF1 pathway, mTORC1, AMPK, and SIRT1 [88]. Metformin is rapidly distributed to many tissues following partial absorption, whereas the luminal concentration in the gastrointestinal tract remains high after a single oral dose [89]. Patients with type 2 diabetes have an increased risk of developing AD [90], as insulin has been shown to prevent Aβ oligomer formation in a dose-dependent matter [90]. A 12-year cohort study revealed that metformin supplementation reduced the AD risk in type 2 diabetes patients, with the risk being further reduced when metformin was combined with an antihyperglycemic agent, sulfonylurea [91]. In contrast, a case-control study revealed that long-term metformin-treated type 2 diabetes patients had a slightly higher risk of developing AD [92]. Despite these contradictory findings, metformin remains a promising CRM, but further research is required to unravel its effects on brain health.

8.4 2DG

2DG is a well-established glycolysis inhibitor first identified by Lane et al. [93] as a potential CRM drug. In this study, rats fed with a 2DG supplemented diet at varying weight-dependent doses revealed that 2DG was toxic at a high dosage, while at the lower dosage, 2DG supplementation had beneficial effects, including reduced blood insulin levels [93]. Rodents maintained on a 2DG-supplemented diet for 2 weeks increased neuronal resistance in AD [94] and PD [95] models. While 7 weeks of 2DG supplementation at a dosage of 0.04% has been shown to attenuate amyloid pathology and increase the levels of BDNF in an AD mouse model [96], toxicity studies revealed that 2DG supplementation at a dosage of 0.2–0.4% may induce cardiotoxicity [97]. 2DG has been linked to the upregulation of CR-related signaling pathways, specifically increased activation of AMPK and SIRT1 [93]. Hence, 2DG remains a viable CRM candidate provided the dose-dependent toxicity can be fully established.

9. Autophagy-inducing agents

Given the cell's declining capacity to sustain efficient autophagic degradation with age, it is not surprising that autophagy dysfunction plays a key role in pathological processes common to aging and neurodegeneration in the elderly [98]. The modulation of autophagic activity may thus be a promising strategy to offset the progression of neurodegenerative processes with age [99]. In addition to adhering to low CR regimes, and the use of CRM drugs, autophagy-induced life extension may also be mediated using the histone acetylase inhibitor, spermidine. Unlike other autophagy-inducing drugs, spermidine has shown no adverse effects during lifelong administration in mice [100], with clinical data indicating good safety and tolerability in elderly subjects during long-term dietary supplementation [101].

9.1 Spermidine

Spermidine is a naturally occurring polyamine that has been shown to decline throughout the aging process in humans [102]. Accordingly, spermidine dietary supplementation in mice (26 weeks) and humans (2 months) has been shown to increase blood polyamine concentrations [103, 104]. Studies reveal that spermidine influences life span, partly, by inducing autophagy through the suppression of E1A-binding protein p300 (EP300), an acetyltransferase that transfers acetyl groups from acetyl coenzyme A to core Atg proteins, thereby inhibiting this pathway [105]. Indeed, He et al. [99] revealed that spermidine's life-extending effects were abolished when autophagy activity was suppressed through *Atg7* or *Beclin1* knockdown *in vivo*, consistent with a causal connection between autophagy induction, neuroprotection, and longevity.

Spermidine's autophagy-inducing potency has been quantified to be equivalent to that of rapamycin [106]. Although dietary supplementation with spermidine has emerged as a promising prevention strategy in aging individuals with an elevated risk of developing AD, the spermidine concentration required for optimal autophagy activity with healthy aging in humans remains unknown. A recent study revealed that spermidine supplementation had no toxic effects even at high concentrations in mice and in older adults at risk for AD [101]. Improved memory performance was reported in the aged subjects after 3 months of spermidine intake compared to the placebo group [107], suggesting that nutritional spermidine may potentially delay memory loss with age.

10. Screening for autophagy-inducing CRMs

Considerable efforts have been made to identify autophagy-inducing drugs which may attenuate the risk for age-associated diseases. Recently, Kaizuka et al. [108] developed an autophagic flux probe which was used to rank

Rank	Drug	GFP/RFP (%)	Pathology	Reference
1	Ciclopirox olamine	17.3	Cancer	Zhou et al. [109]
17	Cladribine (2-CDA)	51.1	AD model	Hayes et al. [110]
27	Sertraline hydrochloride	58.8	Depression	Rainey et al. [111]
29	Loperamide hydrochloride	61.7	Huntington's disease model	Williams et al. [112]
47	Azacitidine	70.0	Hematopoiesis disorders	Abdulhaq and Rossetti [113]

Modified from Kaizuka et al. [108].

Table 1.
Autophagy inducers identified using a sensitive autophagic flux probe.

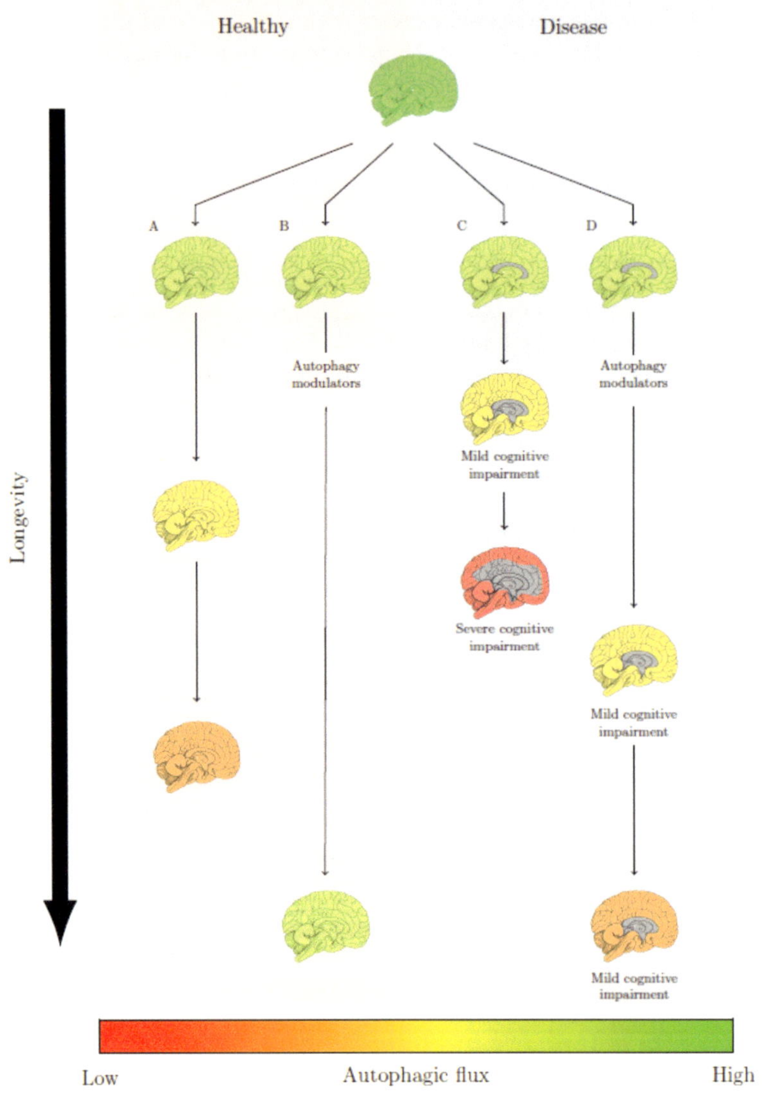

Figure 4.
Matching autophagy induction with autophagic flux decline and dysfunction in brain health and pathology associated with cognitive impairment.

autophagy-inducing drugs according to their level of potency by screening an approved drug library. The autophagic flux probe, i.e., GFP-LC3-RFP-LC3ΔG, is a fusion protein consisting of GFP-LC3 and RFP-LC3, with the C-terminal glycine of RFP-LC3 being deleted. An equal amount of GFP-LC3 and RFP-LC3ΔG is generated in the cytosol, and upon autophagy induction, GFP-LC3 is degraded within autolysosomes, while RFP-LC3ΔG remains in the cytosol and serves as an internal control. GFP-LC3-RFP-LC3ΔG-expressing cells were treated with candidate drugs at varying concentrations for 24 hrs under both nutrient-rich and starvation conditions. The resulting GFP/RFP signal ratio was measured using a microplate reader, with a low GFP/RFP ratio indicating a robust autophagy inducer (**Table 1**). Caution is recommended during cell transfection, as homologous recombination can occur between the two LC3 proteins of the probe. Thus, the isolation of properly expressing GFP-LC3-RFP is recommended. Expression levels of the probe may also vary among different cells/tissues; thus, cells/tissues with similar RFP expression levels should be compared. Lastly, the probe has a relatively low time resolution, making it more ideal for the detection of basal autophagy [108].

Of the 47 autophagy inducers identified, 3 were of relevance to neuroprotection. Importantly, these data indicate firstly, that autophagy activity can be measured accurately and hence standardized and, secondly, that neuronal autophagy decline in aging or neurodegeneration may be matched with an autophagy inducer that is suitable to offset autophagy dysfunction at the respective levels of autophagy activity (**Figure 4**). Further studies using these drugs in the context of healthy brain aging as well as AD pathology are required.

Other antiaging nutrients identified to date, including antioxidants (vitamins A, C, D, and E; quercetin; and coenzyme Q10), and phytochemicals, such as curcumin and epigallocatechin-3-gallate, have been shown to enhance autophagy activity [114]. However, there is a paucity of studies on their overall health benefits in humans.

11. Healthier dietary patterns for successful aging?

Research on the "nutrition transition" reveal that urban areas of developing north and sub-Saharan African countries, Asia, Latin America, and the Middle East share similar dietary pattern shifts [115]. One commonality of this shift is the increased consumption of fat and sugar-laden foods associated with increased risk for age-associated and lifestyle-based diseases. The consumption of nutritionally dense CRM foods, such as marine-based carotenoid-rich food, sweet potatoes, legumes, low-GI grains, fruits, and various flavonoids used in the Okinawan diet, is thought to be the most beneficial food choices for successful aging [48].

12. Future considerations for successful brain aging

Should we restrict our calories/frequently consume CRMs in order to preserve brain health and maintain a sufficiently high neuronal autophagic flux with age? Cumulative evidence from over 70 years of CR research provides compelling support for the role of CR-induced autophagic activity in brain health and longevity [116]. Therefore, a CR regime, alone or in combination with the dietary supplementation of a potent autophagy-inducing CRM, could contribute substantially to successful brain aging, delaying the onset of detrimental effects associated with neuronal proteotoxicity.

Acknowledgements

The authors acknowledge financial support from the South African National Research Foundation (NRF), the South African Medical Research Council (SAMRC), and the Cancer Association of South Africa (CANSA).

Author details

Claudia Ntsapi, Andre du Toit and Ben Loos*
Department of Physiological Sciences, Faculty of Natural Sciences, University of Stellenbosch, Stellenbosch, South Africa

*Address all correspondence to: bloos@sun.ac.za

References

[1] Bloom DE, Chatterji S, et al. Macroeconomic implications of population ageing and selected policy responses. The Lancet. 2015;**385**(9968):649-657

[2] Lopreite M, Mauro M. The effects of population ageing on health care expenditure: A Bayesian VAR analysis using data from Italy. Health Policy (Amsterdam, Netherlands). 2017;**121**(6):663-674

[3] Hebert LE, Weuve J, et al. Alzheimer disease in the United States (2010-2050) estimated using the 2010 census. Neurology. 2013;**80**(19):1778-1783

[4] Sabuncu MR, Desikan RS, et al. The dynamics of cortical and hippocampal atrophy in Alzheimer disease. Archives of Neurology. 2011;**68**(8):1040-1048

[5] Behrens S, Rattinger GB, et al. Use of FDA approved medications for Alzheimer's disease in mild dementia is associated with reduced informal costs of care. International Psychogeriatrics. 2018;**30**(10):1499-1507

[6] Blennow K, Hampel H, et al. Cerebrospinal fluid and plasma biomarkers in Alzheimer disease. Nature Reviews. Neurology. 2010;**6**(3):131-144

[7] Hardy J, Selkoe DJ. The amyloid hypothesis of Alzheimer's disease: Progress and problems on the road to therapeutics. Science. 2002;**297**(5580):353-356

[8] Saito T, Suemoto T, et al. Potent amyloidogenicity and pathogenicity of Aβ43. Nature Neuroscience. 2011;**14**(8):1023-1032

[9] Spillantini MG, Crowther RA, et al. Alpha-Synuclein in filamentous inclusions of Lewy bodies from Parkinson's disease and dementia with lewy bodies. Proceedings of the National Academy of Sciences of the United States of America. 1998;**95**(11):6469-6473

[10] Xilouri M, Brekk OR, et al. Alpha-Synuclein and protein degradation systems: A reciprocal relationship. Molecular Neurobiology. 2013;**47**(2):537-551

[11] Correia SC, Resende R, et al. Alzheimer's disease-related misfolded proteins and dysfunctional organelles on autophagy menu. DNA and Cell Biology. 2015;**34**(4):261-273

[12] Vellai T, Takács-Vellai K, et al. The regulation of aging: Does autophagy underlie longevity? Trends in Cell Biology. 2009;**19**(10):487-494

[13] Kroemer G, Mariño G, et al. Autophagy and the integrated stress response. Molecular Cell. 2010;**40**(2):280-293

[14] Scrivo A, Bourdenx M, et al. Selective autophagy as a potential therapeutic target for neurodegenerative disorders. Lancet Neurology. 2018;**17**(9):802-815

[15] Li W, Li J, Bao J. Microautophagy: Lesser-known self-eating. Cellular and Molecular Life Sciences. 2012;**69**(7):1125-1136

[16] Kaushik S, Cuervo AM. The coming of age of chaperone-mediated autophagy. Nature Reviews. Molecular Cell Biology. 2018;**19**(6):365-381

[17] Mizushima N, Yoshimori T, et al. The role of Atg proteins in autophagosome formation. Annual Review of Cell and Developmental Biology. 2011;**27**:107-132

[18] Ravikumar B, Moreau K, et al. Plasma membrane contributes to the formation of pre-autophagosomal

structures. Nature Cell Biology. 2010;**12**(8):747-757

[19] Klionsky DJ, Abdelmohsen K, et al. Guidelines for the use and interpretation of assays for monitoring autophagy (3rd edition). Autophagy. 2016;**12**(1):1-222

[20] Loos B, du Toit A, J-HS H. Defining and measuring autophagosome flux—Concept and reality. Autophagy. 2014;**10**(11):2087-2096

[21] Jhanwar-Uniyal M, Amin AG, et al. Discrete signaling mechanisms of mTORC1 and mTORC2: Connected yet apart in cellular and molecular aspects. Advances in Biological Regulation. 2017;**64**:39-48

[22] Inoki K, Li Y, et al. TSC2 is phosphorylated and inhibited by Akt and suppresses mTOR signalling. Nature Cell Biology. 2002;**4**(9):648-657

[23] Ikenoue T, Inoki K, et al. Essential function of TORC2 in PKC and Akt turn motif phosphorylation, maturation and signalling. The EMBO Journal. 2008;**27**(14):1919-1931

[24] Medina DL, Settembre C, et al. Methods to monitor and manipulate TFEB activity during autophagy. Methods in Enzymology. 2017;**588**:61-78

[25] Inoki K, Zhu T, et al. TSC2 mediates cellular energy response to control cell growth and survival. Cell. 2003;**115**(5):577-590

[26] Laker R, Drake J, et al. Ampk phosphorylation of Ulk1 is required for targeting of mitochondria to lysosomes in exercise-induced mitophagy. Nature Communications. 2017;**8**(1):548

[27] Lipinski M, Zheng B, et al. Genome-wide analysis reveals mechanisms modulating autophagy in normal brain aging and in Alzheimer's disease. Proceedings of the National Academy of Sciences of the United States of America. 2010;**107**(32):14164-14169

[28] Tóth M, Sigmond T, et al. Longevity pathways converge on autophagy genes to regulate life span in Caenorhabditis elegans. Autophagy. 2008;**4**(3):330-338

[29] Matecic M, Smith D, et al. A microarray-based genetic screen for yeast chronological aging factors. PLoS Genetics. 2010;**6**(4):e1000921

[30] Hara T, Nakamura K, et al. Suppression of basal autophagy in neural cells causes neurodegenerative disease in mice. Nature. 2006;**441**(7095):885-889

[31] Komatsu M, Waguri S, et al. Loss of autophagy in the central nervous system causes neurodegeneration in mice. Nature. 2006;**441**(7095):880-884

[32] Cataldo A, Hamilton D, et al. Properties of the endosomal-lysosomal system in the human central nervous system: Disturbances mark most neurons in populations at risk to degenerate in Alzheimer's disease. Journal of Neuroscience: The Official Journal of the Society for Neuroscience. 1996;**16**(1):186-199

[33] Yu WH, Cuervo AM, et al. Macroautophagy--a novel Beta-amyloid peptide-generating pathway activated in Alzheimer's disease. The Journal of Cell Biology. 2005;**171**(1):87-98

[34] Pickford F, Masliah E, et al. The autophagy-related protein beclin 1 shows reduced expression in early Alzheimer disease and regulates amyloid beta accumulation in mice. The Journal of Clinical Investigation. 2008;**118**(6):2190-2199

[35] Spilman P, Podlutskaya N, et al. Inhibition of mTOR by rapamycin abolishes cognitive deficits and reduces amyloid-beta levels in a mouse model of Alzheimer's disease. PLoS One. 2010;**5**(4):e9979

[36] Majumder S, Richardson A, et al. Inducing autophagy by Rapamycin before, but not after, the formation of plaques and tangles ameliorates cognitive deficits. PLoS One. 2011;**6**(9):e25416

[37] Madeo F, Zimmermann A, et al. Essential role for autophagy in life span extension. The Journal of Clinical Investigation. 2015;**125**(1):85-93

[38] Alirezaei M, Kemball C, et al. Short-term fasting induces profound neuronal autophagy. Autophagy. 2010;**6**(6):702-710

[39] Patterson RE, Laughlin GA, et al. Intermittent fasting and human metabolic health. Journal of the Academy of Nutrition and Dietetics. 2015;**115**(8):1203-1212

[40] Mattson MP. Lifelong brain health is a lifelong challenge: From evolutionary principles to empirical evidence. Ageing Research Reviews. 2015;**20**:37-45

[41] Goodrick CL, Ingram DK, et al. Effects of intermittent feeding upon growth, activity, and life span in rats allowed voluntary exercise. Experimental Aging Research. 1983;**9**(3):203-209

[42] Schafer MJ, Alldred MJ, et al. Reduction of β-amyloid and γ-secretase by calorie restriction in female Tg2576 mice. Neurobiology of Aging. 2015;**36**(3):1293-1302

[43] Halagappa VKM, Guo Z, et al. Intermittent fasting and caloric restriction ameliorate age-related behavioral deficits in the triple-transgenic mouse model of Alzheimer's disease. Neurobiology of Disease. 2007;**26**(1):212-220

[44] Anastasiou CA, Karfopoulou E, et al. Weight regaining: From statistics and behaviors to physiology and metabolism. Metabolism. 2015;**64**(11):1395-1407

[45] Anisimov VN, Popovich IG, et al. Sex differences in aging, life span and spontaneous tumorigenesis in 129/Sv mice neonatally exposed to metformin. Cell Cycle (Georgetown, Tex.). 2015;**14**(1):46-55

[46] Martin B, Pearson M, et al. Sex-dependent metabolic, neuroendocrine, and cognitive responses to dietary energy restriction and excess. Endocrinology. 2007;**148**(9):4318-4333

[47] Rosenbaum MW, Willcox BJ, et al. Okinawa: A Naturally Calorie Restricted Population. Aging and Longevity. Netherlands: Springer; 2010. pp. 43-53

[48] Willcox BJ, Willcox DC, et al. Caloric restriction, the traditional Okinawan diet, and healthy aging: The diet of the world's longest-lived people and its potential impact on morbidity and life span. Annals of the New York Academy of Sciences. 2007;**1114**:434-455

[49] Peters R. Ageing and the brain. Postgraduate Medical Journal. 2006;**82**(964):84-88

[50] Dal-Pan A, Pifferi F, et al. Cognitive performances are selectively enhanced during chronic caloric restriction or resveratrol supplementation in a primate. PLoS One. 2011;**6**(1):e16581

[51] Bondolfi L, Ermini F, et al. Impact of age and caloric restriction on neurogenesis in the dentate gyrus of C57BL/6 mice. Neurobiology of Aging. 2004;**25**(3):333-340

[52] Patel NV, Gordon MN, et al. Caloric restriction attenuates Abeta-deposition in Alzheimer transgenic models. Neurobiology of Aging. 2005;**26**(7):995-1000

[53] Pani G. Neuroprotective effects of dietary restriction: Evidence and mechanisms. Seminars in Cell & Developmental Biology. 2015;**40**:106-114

[54] Nisoli E, Tonello C, et al. Calorie restriction promotes mitochondrial biogenesis by inducing the expression of eNOS. Science. 2005;**310**(5746):314-317

[55] Lee IH, Cao L, et al. A role for the NAD-dependent deacetylase Sirt1 in the regulation of autophagy. Proceedings of the National Academy of Sciences of the United States of America. 2008;**105**(9):3374-3379

[56] Martins R, Lithgow GJ, Link W. Long live FOXO: Unraveling the role of FOXO proteins in aging and longevity. Aging Cell. 2016;**15**(2):196-207

[57] Hardie DG, Ashford MLJ. AMPK: Regulating energy balance at the cellular and whole body levels. Physiology. 2014;**29**(2):99-107

[58] Apfeld J, O'Connor G, et al. The AMP-activated protein kinase AAK-2 links energy levels and insulin-like signals to life span in C. Elegans. Genes & Development. 2004;**18**(24):3004-3009

[59] Cantó C, Jiang L, et al. Interdependence of AMPK and SIRT1 for metabolic adaptation to fasting and exercise in skeletal muscle. Cell Metabolism. 2010;**11**(3, 3):213-219

[60] Kenyon CJ. The genetics of ageing. Nature. 2010;**464**(7288):504-512

[61] Hulbert AJ, Pamplona R, et al. Life and death: Metabolic rate, membrane composition, and life span of animals. Physiological Reviews. 2007;**87**(4):1175-1213

[62] Alers S, Löffler A, et al. Role of AMPK-mTOR-Ulk1/2 in the regulation of autophagy: Cross talk, shortcuts, and feedbacks. Molecular and Cellular Biology. 2012;**32**(1, 1):2-11

[63] Kamada Y, Sekito T, et al. Autophagy in yeast: A TOR-mediated response to nutrient starvation. Current Topics in Microbiology and Immunology. 2004;**279**:73-84

[64] Soare A, Cangemi R, et al. Long-term calorie restriction, but not endurance exercise, lowers core body temperature in humans. Aging. 2011;**3**(4):374-379

[65] Hunt N, Li G, et al. Effect of calorie restriction and refeeding on skin wound healing in the rat. Age (Dordrecht, Netherlands). 2012;**34**(6):1453-1458

[66] Nikolai S, Pallauf K, et al. Energy restriction and potential energy restriction mimetics. Nutrition Research Reviews. 2015;**28**(2):100-120

[67] Bensalem J, Dudonné S, et al. Polyphenols from grape and blueberry improve episodic memory in healthy elderly with lower level of memory performance: A bicentric double-blind, randomized, placebo-controlled clinical study. The Journals of Gerontology. Series A, Biological Sciences and Medical Sciences. 2018

[68] Bensalem J, Dudonné S, et al. Polyphenol-rich extract from grape and blueberry attenuates cognitive decline and improves neuronal function in aged mice. Journal of Nutritional Science. 2018;**7**:e19

[69] Howitz K, Bitterman K, et al. Small molecule activators of sirtuins extend Saccharomyces cerevisiae life span. Nature. 2003;**425**(6954):191-196

[70] Baur J, Pearson K, et al. Resveratrol improves health and survival of mice on a high-calorie diet. Nature. 2006;**444**(7117):337-342

[71] Mattison J, Wang M, et al. Resveratrol prevents high fat/sucrose diet-induced central arterial wall inflammation and stiffening in nonhuman primates. Cell Metabolism. 2014;**20**(1, 1):183-190

[72] Jimenez-Gomez Y, Mattison J, et al. Resveratrol improves adipose insulin signaling and reduces the inflammatory response in adipose tissue of rhesus monkeys on high-fat, high-sugar diet. Cell Metabolism. 2013;**18**(4):533-545

[73] Gambini J, Inglés M, et al. Properties of resveratrol: In vitro and In vivo studies about metabolism, bioavailability, and biological effects in animal models and humans. Oxidative Medicine and Cellular Longevity. 2015;**2015**:837042

[74] Timmers S, Konings E, et al. Calorie restriction-like effects of 30 days of resveratrol supplementation on energy metabolism and metabolic profile in obese humans. Cell Metabolism. 2011;**14**(5):612-622

[75] Poulsen M, Vestergaard P, et al. High-dose resveratrol supplementation in obese men: An investigator-initiated, randomized, placebo-controlled clinical trial of substrate metabolism, insulin sensitivity, and body composition. Diabetes. 2013;**62**(4):1186-1195

[76] Mukherjee S, Ray D, et al. Effects of Longevinex on cardioprotection and its mechanisms of action. Canadian Journal of Physiology and Pharmacology. 2010;**88**(11):1017-1025

[77] Vingtdeux V, Giliberto L, et al. AMP-activated protein kinase signaling activation by resveratrol modulates amyloid-beta peptide metabolism. The Journal of Biological Chemistry. 2010;**285**(12):9100-9113

[78] Turner RS, Thomas R, et al. A randomized, double-blind, placebo-controlled trial of resveratrol for Alzheimer disease. Neurology. 2015;**85**(16):1383-1391

[79] Porquet D, Griñán-Ferré C, et al. Neuroprotective role of trans-resveratrol in a murine model of familial Alzheimer's disease. The Journal of Alzheimer's Disease. 2014;**42**(4):1209-1220

[80] Passtoors W, Beekman M, et al. Gene expression analysis of mTOR pathway: Association with human longevity. Aging Cell. 2013;**12**(1):24-31

[81] Anisimov V, Zabezhinski M, et al. Rapamycin increases life span and inhibits spontaneous tumorigenesis in inbred female mice. Cell Cycle (Georgetown, Tex.). 2011;**10**(24):4230-4236

[82] Cunningham J, Rodgers J, et al. mTOR controls mitochondrial oxidative function through a YY1-PGC-1alpha transcriptional complex. Nature. 2007;**450**(7170):736-740

[83] Majumder S, Caccamo A, et al. Lifelong rapamycin administration ameliorates age-dependent cognitive deficits by reducing IL-1β and enhancing NMDA signaling. Aging Cell. 2012;**11**(2):326-335

[84] Woo H, Chung H, et al. Preclinical evaluation of injectable sirolimus formulated with polymeric nanoparticle for cancer therapy. International Journal of Nanomedicine. 2012;**7**:2197-2208

[85] Samidurai A, Salloum F, et al. Chronic treatment with novel nanoformulated micelles of rapamycin, Rapatar, protects diabetic heart against ischaemia/reperfusion injury. British Journal of Pharmacology. 2017;**174**(24):4771-4784

[86] Comas M, Toshkov I, et al. New nanoformulation of rapamycin Rapatar extends life span in homozygous

p53−/− mice by delaying carcinogenesis. Aging. 2012;**4**(10):715-722

[87] Viollet B, Guigas B, et al. Cellular and molecular mechanisms of metformin: An overview. Clinical Science (London, England: 1979). 2012;**122**(6):253-270

[88] Nelson L, Valentine R, et al. A novel inverse relationship between metformin-triggered AMPK-SIRT1 signaling and p53 protein abundance in high glucose-exposed HepG2 cells. American Journal of Physiology. Cell Physiology. 2012;**303**(1, 1):C4-C13

[89] Foretz M, Guigas B, et al. Metformin: From mechanisms of action to therapies. Cell Metabolism. 2014;**20**(6):953-966

[90] Sridhar G, Lakshmi G, et al. Emerging links between type 2 diabetes and Alzheimer's disease. World Journal of Diabetes. 2015;**6**(5):744-751

[91] Hsu C-C, Wahlqvist M, et al. Incidence of dementia is increased in type 2 diabetes and reduced by the use of sulfonylureas and metformin. The Journal of Alzheimer's Disease. 2011;**24**(3):485-493

[92] Imfeld P, Bodmer M, et al. Metformin, other antidiabetic drugs, and risk of Alzheimer's disease: A population-based case-control study. Journal of the American Geriatrics Society. 2012;**60**(5):916-921

[93] Lane M, Ingram D, Roth GS. 2-Deoxy-D-glucose feeding in rats mimics physiologic effects of calorie restriction. Journal of Anti-Aging Medicine. 1998;**1**(4):327-337

[94] Lee J, Bruce-Keller A, et al. 2-Deoxy-D-glucose protects hippocampal neurons against excitotoxic and oxidative injury: Evidence for the involvement of stress proteins. Journal of Neuroscience Research. 1999;**57**(1, 1):48-61

[95] Duan W, Mattson M. Dietary restriction and 2-deoxyglucose administration improve behavioral outcome and reduce degeneration of dopaminergic neurons in models of Parkinson's disease. Journal of Neuroscience Research. 1999;**57**(2):195-206

[96] Yao J, Chen S, et al. 2-Deoxy-D-glucose treatment induces ketogenesis, sustains mitochondrial function, and reduces pathology in female mouse model of Alzheimer's disease. PLoS One. 2011;**6**(7):e21788

[97] Minor R, Smith D, et al. Chronic ingestion of 2-deoxy-D-glucose induces cardiac vacuolization and increases mortality in rats. Toxicology and Applied Pharmacology. 2010;**243**(3):332-339

[98] Martinez-Lopez N, Athonvarangkul D, et al. Autophagy and aging. Advances in Experimental Medicine and Biology. 2015;**847**:73-87

[99] He L, Lu J, Yue Z. Autophagy in ageing and ageing-associated diseases. Acta Pharmacologica Sinica. 2013;**34**(5):605-611

[100] Eisenberg T, Abdellatif M, et al. Cardioprotection and life span extension by the natural polyamine spermidine. Nature Medicine. 2016;**22**(12):1428-1438

[101] Schwarz C, Stekovic S, et al. Safety and tolerability of spermidine supplementation in mice and older adults with subjective cognitive decline. Aging. 2018;**10**(1):19-33

[102] Eisenberg T, Knauer H, et al. Induction of autophagy by spermidine promotes longevity. Nature Cell Biology. 2009;**11**(11):1305-1314

[103] Soda K, Dobashi Y, et al. Polyamine-rich food decreases age-associated pathology and mortality in

aged mice. Experimental Gerontology. 2009;**44**(11):727-732

[104] Soda K, Kano Y, et al. Increased polyamine intake inhibits age-associated alteration in global DNA methylation and 1,2-dimethylhydrazine-induced tumorigenesis. PLoS One. 2013;**8**(5):e64357

[105] Eisenberg T, Schroeder S, et al. A histone point mutation that switches on autophagy. Autophagy. 2014;**10**(6):1143-1145

[106] du Toit A, Hofmeyr J-HS, Gniadek TJ, Loos B. Measuring autophagosome flux. Autophagy. 2018;**14**(6):1060-1071

[107] Wirth M, Benson G, et al. The effect of spermidine on memory performance in older adults at risk for dementia: A randomized controlled trial. Cortex: A Journal Devoted to the Study of the Nervous System and Behavior. 2018;**109**:181-188

[108] Kaizuka T, Morishita H, et al. An Autophagic flux probe that releases an internal control. Molecular Cell. 2016;**64**(4):835-849

[109] Zhou H, Shang C, et al. Ciclopirox Olamine inhibits mTORC1 signaling by activation of AMPK. Biochemical Pharmacology. 2016;**116**:39-50

[110] Hayes C, Dey D, et al. Chronic Cladribine administration increases amyloid Beta peptide generation and plaque burden in mice. PLoS One. 2012;7(10)

[111] Rainey M, Korostyshevsky D, et al. The antidepressant sertraline targets intracellular Vesiculogenic membranes in yeast. Genetics. 2010;**185**(4):1221-1233

[112] Williams A, Sarkar S, et al. Novel targets for Huntington's disease in an mTOR-independent autophagy pathway. Nature Chemical Biology. 2008;**4**(5):295-305

[113] Abdulhaq H, Rossetti J. The role of azacitidine in the treatment of myelodysplastic syndromes. Expert Opinion on Investigational Drugs. 2007;**16**(12):1967-1975

[114] Cătană C-S, Atanasov A, et al. Natural products with anti-aging potential: Affected targets and molecular mechanisms. Biotechnology Advances. 2018;**36**(6):1649-1656

[115] Popkin B, Adair LS, et al. Global nutrition transition and the pandemic of obesity in developing countries. Nutrition Reviews. 2012;**70**(1):3-21

[116] Mattison J, Vaughan K. An overview of nonhuman primates in aging research. Experimental Gerontology. 2017;**94**:41-45

Section 5

Brain-Visceral Interactions in Enteral Feeding

Chapter 5

Enteral Feeding: Brain-Visceral Interactions in the Processing of Nutrients

María Angeles Zafra Palma, Javier Mahía, María J. Simón, Filomena Molina and Amadeo Puerto

Abstract

Enteral nutrition is often mandatory, especially for patients in vegetative or minimally conscious state. However, its application is nonviable in certain cases due to various adverse effects. Some of these are explained by absence of the cephalic phase of digestion, during which exocrine, endocrine, and motor physiological responses prepare the digestive system to receive, digest, transform, and utilize ingested nutrients. These responses result from the stimulation by nutrients of cephalic sensory systems, mainly in the oropharyngeal cavity, and can also be elicited by food-related thoughts or expectations. The digestive system appears able to rapidly assess the suitability of food and transmit this information to the brain. The vagus nerve and its brainstem relays in the caudal nucleus of the solitary tract (NST) and parabrachial complex appear to participate in the anatomic pathway responsible for this rapid processing. Thus, blockade of the vagus nerve, NST, or external lateral parabrachial region (LPBe) interrupts expression of conditioned taste preferences induced by administration of "predigested" food, while LPBe activation by electric stimulation generates similar preferences to those observed after cephalic food administration. This review may help design enteral diets better adapted to digestive physiology and develop pharmacological interventions against adverse effects of enteral nutrition.

Keywords: enteral nutrition, cephalic phase, rapid processing of nutrients, vagus nerve, gelatinous subnucleus, external lateral parabrachial subnucleus

1. Introduction

Clinical nutrition refers to practices for supplying nutrients to individuals when oral administration is inadvisable, insufficient, or impossible [1]. These are essential to maintain the function of vital organs and systems, minimizing the effects of food deprivation and avoiding nutritional deficiencies [2]. In general, these techniques are divided between enteral nutrition, in which liquid diet is directly administered into the gastric or intestinal cavity, and parenteral nutrition, in which nutritional solutions are delivered intravenously (**Figure 1**; [3]).

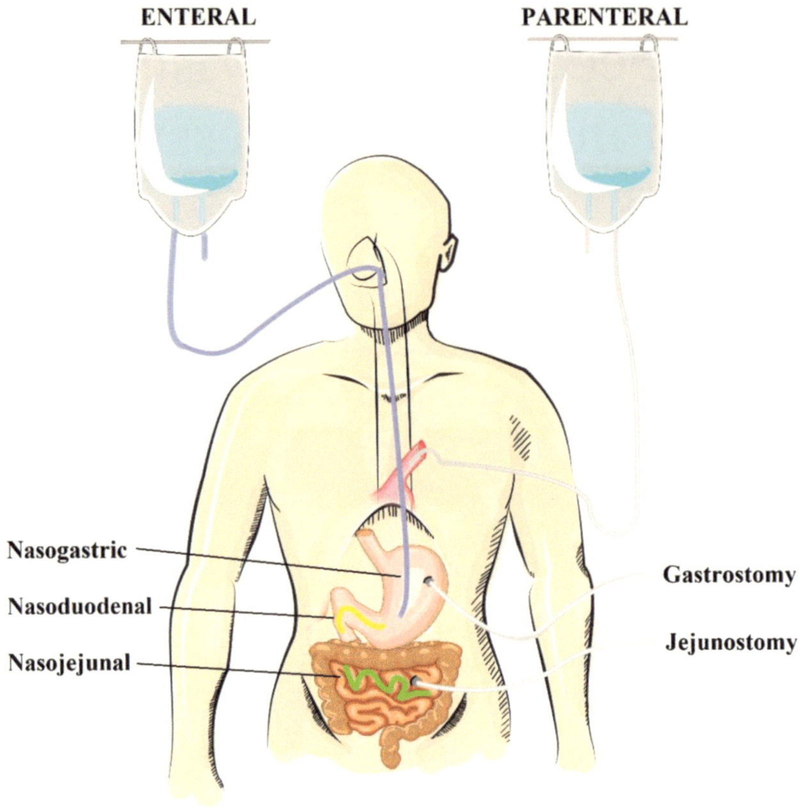

Figure 1.
Enteral (nasogastric, nasoduodenal, nasojejunal, gastrostomy, jejunostomy) and parenteral nutrition.

2. Enteral *versus* parenteral nutrition

Most clinical nutrition specialists report that enteral nutrition has multiple advantages over parental nutrition and should be selected whenever the gastrointestinal tract can be used [3–8]. Parenteral nutrition is more expensive [6, 7, 9] and is usually more invasive in comparison to enteral nutrition, exposing patients to greater risks [10]. Notably, there are important clinical reasons for preferring the enteral administration route because of the association of parenteral nutrition with severe complications, including thromboembolism, severe metabolic fluctuations, hyper- or hypoglycemia, hyperlipidemia, blood electrolyte abnormalities, infectious complications [2, 7, 11, 12], and, more controversially [13], a greater risk of "bacterial translocation" [12, 14–17].

Bacterial translocation takes place when bacteria usually confined to the digestive tract penetrate the intestinal mucosa and invade the lymphatic system, blood system, and numerous internal organs [16–18]. This event has been described as one of the main causes of septicemia and as a risk factor for the onset and progression of multiple organ failure, characterized by the uncontrolled systemic inflammation of internal organs [14, 16, 18–20]. The main factors proposed as possible triggers for bacterial translocation include intestinal mucosal barrier break (increased mucosa permeability), intestinal microflora alteration (bacterial overgrowth), and immune system impairment [5, 17, 18, 21]. These changes are associated with parenteral but not enteral nutrition [21–24].

Under normal conditions, the gastrointestinal mucosa acts as an effective barrier against the migration of microorganisms into the systemic circulation [16, 21, 25]. The integrity of this barrier is determined by the renewal of epithelial cells that compose it and by the number and type of bacteria that it contains [20, 25, 26]. A key stimulus for mucosal cell proliferation and the maintenance of bacterial homeostasis appears to be the presence and availability of nutrients in the intestinal lumen [4–6, 16, 24–27]. The food itself and the hormones released in its presence exert trophic effects on mucosa throughout the gastrointestinal system, from the stomach, small intestine, and colon to the gallbladder and pancreas [5, 24–26]. Both stimuli preserve the intestinal flora [5, 6, 20–22], which in turn critically modulate the immune response by producing the enzymes needed to release immunostimulant nutrients and by activating the secretion of cytokine-like molecules known as bacteriocins [23, 25, 28].

Hence, mucosa atrophy is favored when the gastrointestinal system is not used, as in patients receiving parenteral nutrition. This increases the risk of septic complications [12, 20, 25] and compromises intestinal immunocompetence, because the expression and induction of specific immune responses critically depend on the local microenvironment [20, 25, 28]. These problems are less frequently encountered in patients receiving enteral nutrition [9, 12, 20, 21].

For these reasons, enteral (rather than parenteral) nutrition is recommended in a wide range of clinical situations, including organ transplantation [11], cancer [29], pancreatitis [3, 30], Crohn's disease [31], intestinal resection or inflammation [5], critical disease [3, 6, 7, 9], and the postoperative period [3, 8, 11, 23]. It is also preferred for premature or low-birth-weight infants [12, 32], for the elderly, for neurological patients [29, 33–35], for patients with anorexia nervosa [29], and for those with AIDS [36]. Nevertheless, enteral nutrition is not free of drawbacks, as discussed below [1, 22].

3. Problems associated with enteral nutrition

There is a consensus among health-care professionals that the nutritional status of patients is lower in those receiving enteral nutrition than in those fed orally. Enteral feeding has been associated with several disorders, although it is sometimes difficult to establish whether they are caused by the disease, the specific diet, or by the food administration route [1].

However, regardless of their disease, patients on enteral nutrition often show a series of "secondary" symptoms that can be described as gastrointestinal tract reactions to diet administration, including: pain, discomfort, gastric residual volume, delayed gastric emptying, abdominal bloating and cramps, nausea/vomiting, diarrhea [1, 4, 8, 9, 12, 20, 22, 32, 33–39], metabolic disorders [1, 12], and, when the enteral nutrition is longer term, ulcers and major weight loss [33, 34]. In addition, some patients are unable to tolerate enteral nutrition [9, 22], especially pediatric patients [38, 39].

The causes of these problems have not been fully elucidated, although some psychobiological studies, mainly in animals, have suggested that they may in part result from the entry of food into the digestive tract in "nonphysiological" conditions [40, 41]. The absence of oral stimulation means that the digestive system is not prepared to receive the food (with the appropriate endocrine and exocrine secretions or motor activity changes, etc.), hampering the optimal digestion, absorption, and utilization of the nutrients (see below).

4. Animal models of enteral nutrition: intragastric feeding

In experimental studies, enteral nutrition is known as intragastric or intraintestinal feeding and also appears to be accompanied by numerous disorders that affect the digestion, absorption, and metabolism of nutrients. In these feeding modalities, meals are directly delivered to the gastric cavity (intragastric feeding) or lower segments of the digestive tube, such as the duodenum or jejune (intraintestinal feeding), generally using a permanently implanted catheter. A physiological variable or function is then studied and compared with results obtained for oral feeding or for sham feeding, in which the food is orally ingested but extracted *via* a cannula before reaching the stomach.

One of the first authors to document alterations in animals caused by intragastric feeding was the Russian scientist Ivan Pavlov [42], whose studies masterfully demonstrated the marked importance of the passage of food through oropharyngeal systems for its subsequent digestion [43, 44]. This oropharyngeal stimulation, designated "psychic reflex" by Pavlov, is now known as the cephalic phase of digestion, which comprises a set of autonomic and endocrinal responses to stimulation by the food of sensory perceptive systems in the head and particularly in the oropharyngeal cavity. Nevertheless, although these cephalic responses are preferentially initiated by contact with the food, they can also be effectively elicited just by seeing or anticipating it or by thoughts or any learned cues associated with it [40, 42, 44].

The digestive events triggered by cephalic stimulation are mediated by vagal parasympathetic efferents except for salivary secretions, which are partly controlled by sympathetic and nonvagal parasympathetic fibers. These vagal efferents, which are distributed throughout the digestive tube and associated digestive organs (liver, pancreas, and gallbladder), largely originate in the dorsal motor nucleus of the vagus (DMV), which is localized in the caudal medulla oblongata close to the floor of the fourth ventricle and is closely related to the nucleus of the solitary tract, the main structure receiving visceral signals from the digestive system [40–44].

DMV activity is directly or indirectly modulated by centers at upper levels of the nervous system that are responsible for the changes in digestive function that take place during the cephalic phase of digestion. This descending control of the DMV has been reported for such structures as the insular cortex, medial prefrontal cortex, central nucleus of the amygdala, bed nucleus of the stria terminalis, tegmental ventral area, and nucleus accumbens. Many of these signals reach the DMV through relays in hypothalamic regions (posterior hypothalamus and paraventricular nucleus) and brainstem regions (e.g., periaqueductal gray matter or parabrachial nucleus) [40, 44–47].

Pavlov reported that when food was directly introduced into the stomach, the secretion of gastric juices was delayed and scant, with weak digestive power, contrasting with the rapid and abundant cascade of gastric secretions observed when the same nutrients passed through the oropharyngeal cavity after their real or sham intake. He concluded that the low gastric juice secretion in enteral nutrition delays and considerably prolongs digestion [42].

The absence of oropharyngeal stimulation also indirectly delays other digestive secretions. It was reported by Pavlov that intragastrically administered food is not accompanied by salivary secretions, whose arrival in the stomach cavity stimulates the release of gastric juices [42]. It has also been demonstrated that the digestion of carbohydrates and fats that starts in the mouth through the action of salivary amylase and lipase continues in the stomach [48–50]. Hence, the absence of saliva delays gastric secretion and hampers the digestion of some nutrients. There is also an indirect effect on the release of pancreatic juices, whose secretion is determined by the level of hydrochloric acid in the stomach [42].

Absence of the cephalic phase impacts on digestion-related substances throughout the digestive system, from the mouth or stomach (e.g., salivary enzymes, hydrochloric acid, gastrin, pepsinogen, immunoglobulins, etc.), as mentioned above, to the small intestine (bicarbonate or digestive enzymes), liver, or pancreas (numerous hormones) (for review, see references [40, 44]). Many secretions triggered by cephalic stimulation are also specific and adapted to the nature of the food [42, 51–56]. In other words, food components appear to be identified before they reach the stomach, allowing the digestive system to be specifically prepared for their transformation and utilization [40, 57].

Removal of the cephalic phase affects not only endocrine and exocrine secretions but also gastrointestinal motor activity, with an anticipatory increase in cephalic stimulation [58–61]. The intragastric feeding of experimental animals has also been found to markedly accelerate the outflow of gastric contents into the duodenum [62–64], which might be responsible for the discomfort experienced by patients with "dumping syndrome" [62]. This syndrome is observed in humans who have undergone abdominal vagotomy and is characterized by the rapid emptying of gastric contents into the duodenum, producing nausea and epigastric pain [65]. In this regard, the intraintestinal administration of nutrients (fats) was found to significantly damage the intestinal mucosa [63, 66].

Disorders induced by the absence of oropharyngeal stimulation extend to postabsorptive stages [54, 57, 62, 64, 67–70]. In human studies, glucose intolerance (increased blood levels) and reduced blood glucagon levels were observed after intragastric glucose administration, but not when this was accompanied by oral sensory stimulation through modified sham feeding [71]. It has also been demonstrated that lipolysis is slower with intragastric *versus* oral feeding, leading to higher plasma levels of fatty acids [62].

Responses that are affected by the absence of cephalic stimulation can be observed in other levels of the digestive system and beyond, including postprandial thermogenesis, anticipatory rise in heart rate, increased respiratory rate in response to eating, and changes in the transport and intestinal absorption of nutrients and in bile flow and secretin release, among others [49, 72–75].

Taken together, published studies confirm that the cephalic phase not only optimizes food digestion but also intervenes in processes related to nutrient absorption and metabolism. Many of these effects may be secondary to the release of gastrointestinal hormones, whose secretion is stimulated by the anticipation and presence of food in the oropharyngeal cavity [76–79].

5. Is intragastric feeding stressful?

According to the above-reported studies, intragastric or intraintestinal feeding means that the digestive system is not prepared to receive, digest, process, or even appropriately utilize the administered nutrients. They would arrive in the system under nonphysiological, negative conditions, which may in part account for the digestive problems that can often make enteral nutrition nonviable.

Taste learning is one of the behavioral procedures used by scientists to determine whether individuals perceive the food reaching the digestive system as positive or negative. In these learning tasks, two nonnutritional flavored solutions of water are offered, with the intragastric/intraintestinal administration of a nutritional stimulus being associated with one solution and of an innocuous, nonnutritional stimulus (e.g., physiological saline) with the other. The preference of animals is determined after multiple sessions pairing the taste and visceral stimuli [80–83].

Studies using this technique have demonstrated that the direct administration of complex food into the gastric cavity is a powerful way to establish flavor-conditioned aversions [66, 80, 84–86]. Thus, when rats were subjected to a discriminative flavor learning task using whole milk as visceral stimulus, they preferred the flavor associated with physiological saline and strongly rejected the flavor associated with the food, even after a 22-h food deprivation period [80, 84–86]. Similar results were observed with intraintestinal feeding, finding that association of the intraduodenal administration of fats or glucose with the oral intake of saccharose or water produced a strong rejection of both in subsequent presentations [66, 80, 81, 86–88].

Results obtained with the enteral administration of natural food markedly contrast with those obtained for the intragastric administration of food subjected to cephalic processing (aspirated from the stomachs of donor subjects shortly after its oral consumption). Unlike observations with natural food, the animals developed a strong preference for the taste stimulus associated with the administration of "predigested" food and rejected the stimulus associated with physiological saline [80, 81, 86–88]. Hence, enterally administered foods are experienced as rewarding/positive when they have undergone oropharyngeal processing, and assistance of the cephalic phase appears to adapt enteral diets more closely to digestive physiology. According to these data, the digestive system also seems perfectly prepared for the rapid assessment of the suitability of foods and for the transmission of this information to the central nervous system.

Results of research in animals have prompted numerous clinical studies. Although enteral nutrition was not a routine clinical practice until the 1960s, food had long been administered *via* gastric catheters, with the first case being published in 1564 by Matthew Cornax, a Viennese professor and physician. The first reports on gastric function and disorders in individuals fed *via* gastric catheters were presented by Coronel William Beaumont (1833) and the French physician Charles Richet (1879), who described the appearance of reddish blemishes and spots, scabs, and fragments of gastric mucosa, as well as delays in digestion and gastric emptying [89].

One of the most famous studies in this field was published by Wolf and Wolff and known as "Tom's case." In 1895, at the age of 9 years, Tom underwent gastronomy after accidentally eating boiling food and was only able to consume food *via* gastric catheter for the next 65 years. Tom was studied by various authors during this time, and one of the main findings was that digestion was not optimal when the food was deposited directly in the stomach and the intake was wholly unsatisfactory, leading to his malnourishment. However, when he was allowed to taste and chew the food before intragastric administration, at his own request, he gained weight and developed a good appetite [90]. Other similar reports in the literature include the case of a 24-year-old woman presented during the Annual Meeting of the American College of Gastroenterology in 1950 [91] and of a patient with a 29-year history of complete esophageal obstruction and large permanent gastrostomy [92], who both acquired the habit of tasting and partially chewing food before intragastric administration. Although we have been unable to trace more recent studies of this type, other results obtained in humans have highlighted the importance of cephalic stimulation in nutrition. For instance, oral stimulation with monosodium glutamate (flavor enhancer that improves taste/palatability and augments salivary flow) increased the appetite and weight of elderly patients with problems of taste sensitivity, appetite loss, and weight loss, improving their overall health [93, 94]. Similar findings were reported in neonates with established enteral feeding, whose discomfort was reduced by oral stimulation with glucose [95], and in restrained eaters, whose food intake was increased by the sensory experience of tasting fat [96].

In summary, these data indicate that the signals produced by food in the oropharyngeal cavity trigger a cascade of exocrine, endocrine, and motor reactions that prepare the digestive system for the reception, digestion, absorption, and metabolism of the food ingested, allowing feeding to be perceived as a satisfactory or rewarding event. When these signals are missing, a series of noxious consequences can hamper the adequate development of these processes, making the feeding experience negative or "stressful" [40, 41, 44, 62].

It is therefore possible that some of the noxious effects of enteral nutrition can be palliated by administering diets that imitate "cephalic" food in some way. This possibility is currently under investigation in our laboratory.

6. Transmission pathways of rewarding visceral information to the central nervous system

In general, two distinct procedures can be used to establish flavor learning, designated by our group as concurrent and sequential flavor learning. Two nonnutritional flavored stimuli with their respective intragastric administrations are simultaneously offered during a short time period (usually 7 min) in concurrent learning, whereas the stimuli are presented in alternating sessions in sequential learning (**Figure 2**). A key difference between these procedures is that animals must detect and process visceral stimuli very quickly to establish an association in concurrent learning, whereas this can be established in a more delayed fashion in sequential learning [82, 93, 88].

Using these procedures, and with the aim of being able to palliate the negative effects of enteral nutrition in the future, our group has studied the rapid pathway for processing information related to nutritional stimuli present in the gastrointestinal tract (concurrent learning), especially in the case of suitable or rewarding ("cephalic") foods [81, 87, 88].

Information from the gastrointestinal tract reaches the brain *via* complementary humoral and neural pathways [97]. However, given the aforementioned time constraints of concurrent taste, participation of the humoral pathway in this task appears unlikely, and the neural pathway would be responsible for the transmission of information under these learning conditions [87].

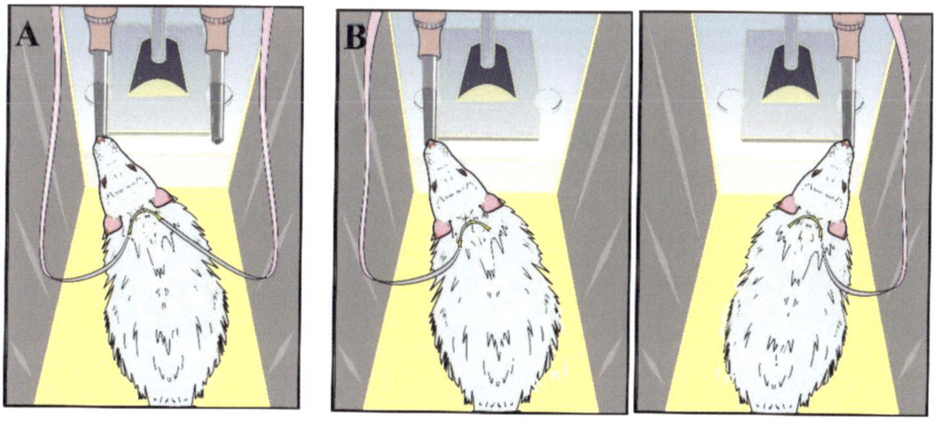

Figure 2.
Experimental procedure followed in concurrent (A) and sequential (B) flavor learning. In the former, two flavored stimuli are presented at the same time; when the animal voluntarily consumes one of these stimuli, it is simultaneously and intragastrically administered with the associated visceral stimulus (e.g., predigested nutrients through an intragastric cannula); when the animal consumes the other stimulus, it is simultaneously and intragastrically administered with the other visceral product (e.g., physiological saline) through a second cannula. The same procedure is followed in sequential learning (B) except that each of the flavored stimuli and their respective intragastric administrations are presented in alternate sessions.

Neuroanatomical and neurophysiological studies have demonstrated that the gastrointestinal tract receives both vagal and spinal nerve fibers [97], and either may have carried nutritional information to the brain in our studies. However, numerous physiological and behavioral investigations have indicated that spinal visceral afferents are less important in nutrition [98] and appear more related to nociceptive processes [99]. For this reason, we have focused on the vagal system in our experiments on the neural substrates involved in transmitting rewarding visceral information to the central nervous system.

Vagal afferents are distributed throughout the digestive system (**Figure 3**) and receive detailed information on the specific nature of the nutrients present in the gastrointestinal lumen *via* interoceptors (chemo-, osmo-, thermo-, and mechanoreceptors) [97, 100, 101]. This takes place directly, through the free diffusion of luminal chemicals across epithelial cells, and also indirectly *via* paracrine messengers released by enteroendocrine cells, which act as sensory transducers ("taste" cells)

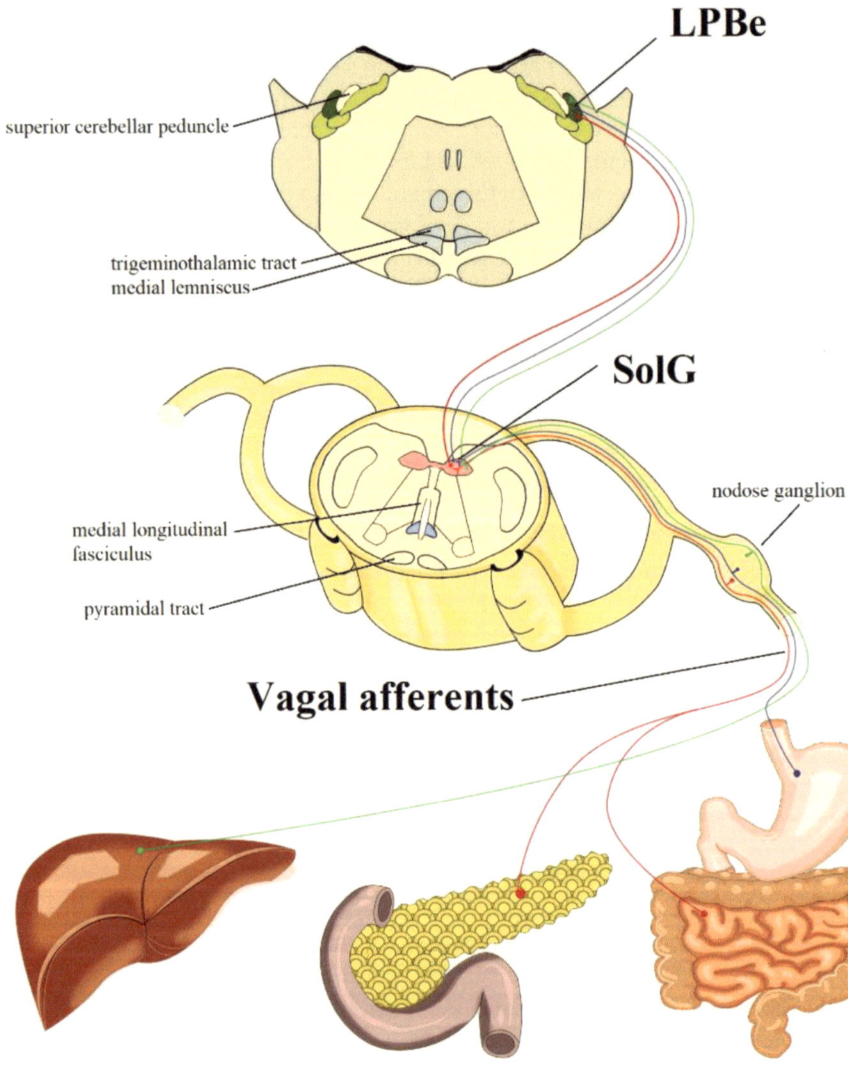

Figure 3.
Anatomical pathways and nuclei involved in the rapid detection and processing of nutritional rewarding visceral information (SolG: gelatinous subnucleus of nucleus of solitary tract; LPBe: external lateral parabrachial subnucleus).

that detect the physical and chemical nature of luminal contents [100, 102–104]. Vagal afferents with nutritional information ascend toward the brain in parallel with autonomic motor fibers, forming bundles on both sides of the esophagus and ending in the nodose ganglion, from which central vagal branches extend toward their first brain relay: the nucleus of the solitary tract (NST) [105–106].

In rats, the NTS is a small-sized bilateral structure that ends in a single midline nucleus caudal to the area postrema (AP), one of the main circumventricular organs of the brain (Y-shaped in horizontal plane). Three regions have been differentiated in the anteroposterior dimension of the NTS: a rostral region that extends from the rostral pole of the nucleus to the point where the medial division contacts the fourth ventricle border; an intermediate band that extends from this last point to the caudal end of the AP; and a caudal division wholly occupied by the commissural sub-nucleus [105–107]. Most of the subnuclei of the NTS are found in its intermediate region, especially in the medial division (localized medially to the solitary tract, a bundle of fibers that crosses the entire anteroposterior extent of the nucleus) [107].

The NTS is the first relay for a wide range of special and general visceral afferent sensory fibers (oropharyngeal, gastrointestinal, cardiovascular, and respiratory), which are relatively segregated in subnuclei distributed throughout its rostrocaudal dimension. Those originating in the gastrointestinal system largely terminate in subnuclei in the medial division of the intermediate-caudal NTS [105–106].

Our group has investigated the participation of vagal afferents in the rapid transmission of rewarding nutritional information to the brain using capsaicin (8-methyl N-vanillyl-6-nonenamide), the pungent component in red pepper of the genus *Capsicum* (family Solanaceae). When topically applied, capsaicin causes the initial excitation of thinly myelinated Aδ- and unmyelinated C afferent fibers (enhancing the release and inhibiting the reuptake of substance P and other neuroactive peptides from terminals), producing a transient hyperalgesia. This is followed by a refractory period with reduced sensitivity, explaining its clinical application to treat different types of pain. After prolonged or repeated exposure, capsaicin produces a permanent degeneration of these fibers and a persistent desensitization. Therefore, perineural application of this substance provides an important neuropharmacological tool for determining the specific role of an afferent pathway [108].

We applied capsaicin around the esophagus, selectively lesioning unmyelinated afferents and weakly myelinated fibers [108], which are both largely present in the vagus nerve [109, 110]. We found that information transmission mediated by capsaicin-sensitive vagal afferents is essential in concurrent taste discrimination tasks [87]. Thus, neurochemical interruption of this pathway hampers the establishment of taste preferences induced by the intragastric administration of "cephalic" foods, which is achieved without difficulty by neurologically intact animals.

However, capsaicin-sensitive afferents are not indispensable for the induction of taste preferences using sequential tasks. In this case, both capsaicin-treated and neurologically intact animals effectively learn the task and show clear preferences for taste stimuli associated with the intragastric administration of predigested nutrients. These results support the idea that information is unlikely to be transmitted to the brain *via* spinal or humoral mechanisms in concurrent tasks, because capsaicin-treated animals could be expected to learn the task if this was the case, and they did not [87]. Because each flavor is presented with its respective intragastric administration on alternate days in the sequential modality, long time periods are available for the detection and processing of the visceral stimuli. Hence, neurologically intact animals could use both neural pathways (likely while the food is present in the gastrointestinal tract) and humoral pathways (after the absorption of nutrients), whereas capsaicin-treated animals could only use the humoral (and/or spinal) pathway, although this would be sufficient to develop the corresponding taste preference behaviors.

Anatomical, physiological, and immunohistochemical studies have demonstrated that vagal afferents from the upper gastrointestinal tract project toward the intermediate-caudal region of the NST (**Figure 3**), a gateway for visceral signal processing [111]. Thus, various subnuclei of the intermediate-caudal region of the NST (NSTic) show c-fos activity after normal food intake [112], after intragastric or intraduodenal nutrient administration [113–115], and in situations of gastric [116] and intestinal [117] distension, among others. In many of these cases, NSTic activation is abolished by the chemical or surgical lesioning of vagal afferents [114, 118].

Given the time constraints implicit in the concurrent procedure, the digestive segments most likely to be involved in this learning modality (i.e., responsible for initial detection of the visceral stimulus) would be proximal ones (preferentially the stomach and duodenum). Sensory visceral information is known to be organized topographically in the NSTic with relative anatomical segregation [105, 106]. For instance, a high density of gastric vagal afferents is concentrated in the lateral portion of the dorsomedial NST in a cell cluster known as the gelatinous nucleus [105–107, 111, 119], whereas afferents from the duodenum and other segments of the small intestine are distributed in different areas of the dorsomedial nucleus, especially in more caudal and medial areas of the intermediate region [105, 106, 117].

Our group recently demonstrated that the gelatinous subnucleus (SolG) participates in the learning of concurrent taste preferences induced by intragastrically administered "cephalic" foods [88]. It therefore appears that the gelatinous nucleus (SolG), alongside capsaicin-sensitive vagal afferents, may participate in the neural pathway that rapidly processes rewarding nutritional information from the upper gastrointestinal tract. This subnucleus almost exclusively concentrates gastric vagal afferents [106, 113, 117, 119] and is a receptor of fine vagal afferents [120], that is, the type of fibers lesioned by capsaicin [108]. In addition, capsaicin-induced damage of small ganglion cells was found to produce axonal degeneration in the SolG, among other regions [121].

The NSTic in turn relays visceral information from the gut to the lateral division of the pontine parabrachial complex (**Figure 3**), especially to its lateral external subnucleus.

The parabrachial complex is a grouping of subnuclei that surround the superior cerebellar peduncle along its course through the dorsolateral pons. In rats, the subnuclei localized dorsally to the peduncle constitute its lateral division (LPB) and those localized ventrally the medial division [122]. The external subnucleus (LPBe), localized at the most lateral border and throughout the rostrocaudal dimension of the LPB, concentrates information from both the stomach and duodenum, receiving a large number of the afferents projected from the dorsomedial NTS, including the SolG[107, 122, 123].

These anatomical connections allow modification of LPBe activity by electrical stimulation of the vagus nerve and by the intragastric administration of various nutrients [114, 124, 125]. Moreover, the intragastric application of nutrients induces c-fos expression in intermediate-caudal and dorsomedial NST subnuclei and in the LPBe, among other regions [114, 115]. This dual activation has also been observed after the administration of substances that positively or negatively affect food intake, including pharmacological agents (such as methyl palmoxirate, 2,5-anhydro-D-mannitol, or dexfenfluramine) and various hormones (e.g., cholecystokinin, bombesin, or secretin) [126–131]. These effects of neuronal activation and/or intake can also be abolished or attenuated by truncal vagotomy or perivagal capsaicin treatment [114, 126, 130–134].

Our laboratory has also addressed the possibility of the LPBe nucleus being part of the rapid processing pathway of rewarding information related to nutrients present in the upper gastrointestinal tract in our laboratory. Unlike neurologically intact animals, LPBe-lesioned animals proved unable to develop taste preferences induced by the intragastric administration of "cephalic or predigested" foods in concurrent taste learning tasks, but both groups were able to learn taste preferences in sequential taste learning tasks [81].

We have also used other procedures to explore the involvement of the LPBe in rewarding processes, including the induction of taste and place preferences by electrical stimulation of this subnucleus [135]. In addition, large lesions of the LPB, including the external subnucleus, appear to reverse aversive effects of the intragastric administration of natural, nonpredigested nutrients, avoiding rejection of the associated taste stimulus and appearing to induce a flavor preference (*versus* water) in late trials of the task [85].

Considered together, these data suggest that the rapid processing of visceral information on rewarding nutrition (in upper gastrointestinal segments) is mediated by a neural pathway that originates peripherally in the vagus nerve and includes NSTic regions (e.g., SolG) and the LPBe [81, 87, 88]. In fact, this visceral vagal-NSTic-LPBe information pathway also appears to participate in other physiological processes requiring the rapid transmission of nutritional information. We recently showed that both the vagus nerve [136] and SolG [137] or LPBe [138] are essential in circumstances that require the immediate adjustment of food intake, extracting part of ingested food immediately after ending a meal and finding that approximately the same amount was reingested by neurologically intact animals but a much smaller amount by lesioned animals.

The vagus nerve-NSTic-LPBe pathway also proved essential for the rapid transmission of nonnutritional visceral information. We found that the vagus nerve [83] and NSTic [139] or LPBe [140] are necessary for concurrent taste aversion learning but not for sequential TAL.

According to the studies presented in this chapter, organisms have at least two complementary neurobiological systems for the detection and processing of nutritional rewarding visceral information: one that depends on the vagus nerve, NSTic, and LPBe, and another that is independent of this pathway. The former appears to participate when rapid information processing is needed and the latter when there are no time constraints.

7. Conclusions

Research into the biological mechanisms underlying nutritional behavior is exhilarating, both for the simple pleasure of unraveling these complex phenomena and for its potential importance in numerous clinical fields, including artificial nutrition. As shown in our review, enteral nutrition for any reason and of any type is frequently associated with adverse effects whose causes have yet to be fully elucidated. Studies by our group suggest that at least some of these negative effects may result from the absence of the cephalic phase of digestion. Further investigations of the physiology of this nutritional process are needed to support the design of enteral diets better adapted to digestive physiology and the development of pharmacological strategies that counteract its noxious effects.

Acknowledgements

The authors are grateful to Richard and Layla Davies for their assistance with the English version of this chapter and to Alejandro Navarro for creating Figures.

Conflict of interest

The authors declared no potential conflicts of interest with respect to the research, authorship, and/or publication of this article.

Author details

María Angeles Zafra Palma[‡*], Javier Mahía[‡], María J. Simón, Filomena Molina and Amadeo Puerto[†]

Department of Psychobiology and Mind, Brain and Behavior Research Center (CIMCYC), University of Granada, Spain

[‡] These two authors contributed equally to the manuscript

[†] In memoriam

*Address all correspondence to: mazafra@ugr.es

References

[1] Meguid MM, Campos AC. Nutritional management of patients with gastrointestinal fistulas. The Surgical Clinic of North America. 1996;**76**(5):1035-1080. DOI: 10.1016/S0039-6109(05)70497-7

[2] Irving SY, Simone SD, Hicks FW, Verger JT. Nutrition for the critically ill child: Enteral and parenteral support. AACN Nurses Clinical Issues. 2000;**11**:541-558. DOI: 10.1097/00044067-200011000-00007

[3] Seres DS, Valcarcel M, Guillaume A. Advantages of enteral nutrition over parenteral nutrition. Therapeutic Advances in Gastroenterology. 2013;**6**(2):157-167. DOI: 10.1177/1756283X12467564

[4] Heymsfield SB, Bethel RA, Ansley JD, Nixon DW, Rudman D. Enteral hyperalimentation: An alternative to central venous hyperalimentation. Annals of Internal Medicine. 1979;**90**(1):63-71. DOI: 10.7326/0003-4819-90-1-63

[5] Jenkins AP, Thompson RP. Enteral nutrition and the small intestine. Gut. 1994;**35**(12):1765-1769. DOI: 10.1136/gut.35.12.1765

[6] Jolliet P, Pichard C, Biolo G, Chioléro R, Grimble G, Leverve X, et al. Enteral nutrition in intensive care patients: A practical approach. Clinical Nutrition. 1999;**18**(1):47-56. DOI: 10.1054/clnu.1998.0001

[7] Gramlich L, Kichian K, Pinilla J, Rodych NJ, Dhaliwal R, Heyland DK. Does enteral nutrition compared to parenteral nutrition result in better outcomes in critically ill adult patients? A systematic review of the literature. Nutrition. 2004;**20**(10):843-848. DOI: 10.1016/j.nut.2004.06.003

[8] Bengmark S. Clinical nutrition. In: Zafra MA, Molina F, Puerto A, editors. The Cephalic/Neural Phase in Nutrition. Kerala: Research Signpost; 2009. pp. 93-116

[9] Huang J, Yang L, Zhuang Y, Qi H, Chen X, Lv K. Current status and influencing factors of barriers to enteral feeding of critically ill patients: A multicenter study. Journal of Clinical Nursing. 2018. DOI: 10.1111/jocn.14667

[10] van de Ven CJ. Nasogastric enteral feeding in hyperemesis gravidarum. The Lancet. 1997;**349**(9050):445-446. DOI: 10.1016/S0140-6736(05)61177-4

[11] Wicks C, Somasundaram S, Bjarnason I, Menzies IS, Routley D, Potter D, et al. Comparison of enteral feeding and total parenteral nutrition after liver transplantation. The Lancet. 1994;**344**(8926):837-840. DOI: 10.1016/S0140-6736(94)92824-X

[12] Finck C. Enteral versus parenteral nutrition in the critically ill. Nutrition. 2000;**16**(5):393-394. DOI: 10.1016/S0899-9007(00)00235-5

[13] MacFie J. Enteral versus parenteral nutrition: The significance of bacterial translocation and gut-barrier function. Nutrition. 2000;**16**(7-8):606-611. DOI: 10.1016/S0899-9007(00)00249-5

[14] Alverdy JC, Aoys E, Moss GS. Total parenteral nutrition promotes bacterial translocation from the gut. Surgery. 1988;**104**(2):185-190

[15] Qiu JG, Delany HM, Teh EL, Freundlich L, Gliedman ML, Steinberg JJ, et al. Contrasting effects of identical nutrients given parenterally or enterally after 70% hepatectomy: Bacterial translocation. Nutrition. 1997;**13**(5):431-437. DOI: 10.1016/S0899-9007(97)91281-8

[16] Anastasilakis CD, Ioannidis O, Gkiomisi AI, Botsios D. Artificial

nutrition and intestinal mucosal barrier functionality. Digestion. 2013;**88**(3):193-208. DOI: 10.1159/000353603

[17] Cahova M, Bratova M, Wohl P. Parenteral nutrition-associated liver disease: The role of the gut microbiota. Nutrients. 2017;**9**(9):E987. DOI: 10.3390/nu9090987

[18] Balzan S, de Almeida Quadros C, de Cleva R, Zilberstein B, Cecconello I. Bacterial translocation: Overview of mechanisms and clinical impact. Journal of Gastroenterology and Hepatology. 2007;**22**(4):464-471. DOI: 10.1111/j.1440-1746.2007.04933.x

[19] Marshall JC, Christou NV, Horn R, Meakins JL. The microbiology of multiple organ failure. The proximal gastrointestinal tract as an occult reservoir of pathogens. Archives of Surgery. 1988;**123**(3). DOI: 309-315. DOI:10.1001/archsurg.1988.01400270043006

[20] Moore FA, Feliciano DV, Andrassy RJ, McArdle AH, Booth FV, Morgenstein-Wagner TB, et al. Early enteral feeding, compared with parenteral, reduces postoperative septic complications. The results of a meta-analysis. Annals of Surgery. 1992;**216**(2):172-183

[21] Lara TM, Jacobs DO. Effect of critical illness and nutritional support on mucosal mass and function. Clinical Nutrition. 1998;**17**(3):99-105. DOI: 10.1016/S0261-5614(98)80002-2

[22] Dive A. Enteral nutrition in the critically ill: Is the gut working properly? Nutrition. 1999;**15**(5):404-405. DOI: 10.1016/S0899-9007(99)00027-1

[23] Sigalet DL, Mackenzie SL, Hameed SM. Enteral nutrition and mucosal immunity: Implications for feeding strategies in surgery and trauma. Canadian Journal of Surgery. 2004;**47**(2):109-116

[24] Barrett M, Demehri FR, Teitelbaum DH. Intestine, immunity, and parenteral nutrition in an era of preferred enteral feeding. Current Opinion in Clinical Nutrition and Metabolic Care. 2015;**18**(5):496-500. DOI: 10.1097/MCO.0000000000000208

[25] McClave SA, Heyland DK. The physiologic response and associated clinical benefits from provision of early enteral nutrition. Nutrition in Clinical Practice. 2009;**24**(3):305-315. DOI: 10.1177/0884533609335176

[26] Johnson LR. Regulation of gastrointestinal mucosal growth. Physiological Reviews. 1988;**68**(2):456-502. DOI: 10.1152/physrev.1988.68.2.456

[27] Shanahan F, van Sinderen D, O'Toole PW, Stanton C. Feeding the microbiota: Transducer of nutrient signals for the host. Gut. 2017;**66**(9):1709-1717. DOI: 10.1136/gutjnl-2017-313872

[28] Bengmark S. Immunonutrition - concluding remarks. Nutrition. 1999;**15**(1):57-61. DOI: 10.1016/S0899-9007(98)00122-1

[29] Bozzetti F. Quality of life and enteral nutrition. Current Opinion in Clinical Nutrition and Metabolic Care. 2008;**11**(5):661-665. DOI: 10.1097/MCO.0b013e32830a7099

[30] Marik PE, Zaloga GP. Meta-analysis of parenteral nutrition versus enteral nutrition in patients with acute pancreatitis. BMJ. 2004;**328**(7453):1407. DOI: 10.1136/bmj.38118.593900.55

[31] Fernández-Bañares F, Cabré E, González-Huix F, Gassull MA. Enteral nutrition as primary therapy in Crohn's disease. Gut. 1994;**35**(Suppl 1):S55-S59. DOI: 10.1136/gut.35.1_Suppl.S55

[32] Li N, Wang W, Wu G, Wang J. Nutritional support for low birth weight infants: Insights from animal studies. The British Journal of Nutrition. 2017;**117**(10):1390-1402. DOI: 10.1017/S000711451700126X

[33] Ciocon JO, Silverstone FA, Graver LM, Foley CJ. Tube feedings in elderly patients. Indications, benefits, and complications. Archives of Internal Medicine. 1988;**148**(2):429-433. DOI: 10.1001/archinte.1988.00380020173022

[34] Henderson CT, Trumbore LS, Mobarhan S, Benya R, Miles TP. Prolonged tube feeding in long-term care: Nutritional status and clinical outcomes. Journal of the American College of Nutrition. 1992;**11**(3):309-325. DOI: 10.1080/07315724.1992.10718232

[35] Punchik B, Komissarov E, Zeldez V, Freud T, Samson T, Press Y. Doctors' knowledge and attitudes regarding enteral feeding and eating problems in advanced dementia. Dementia and Geriatric Cognitive Disorders Extra. 2018;**8**(2):268-276. DOI: 10.1159/000489489

[36] Henderson RA, Saavedra JM, Perman JA, Hutton N, Livingston RA, Yolken RH. Effect of enteral tube feeding on growth of children with symptomatic human immunodeficiency virus infection. Journal of Pediatric Gastroenterology and Nutrition. 1994;**18**(4):429-434

[37] Bastow MD. Complications of enteral nutrition. Gut. 1986;**27**(Suppl 1):51-55. DOI: 10.1136/gut.27.Suppl_1.51

[38] Pahsini K, Marinschek S, Khan Z, Dunitz-Scheer M, Scheer PJ. unintended adverse effects of enteral nutrition support: parental perspective. Journal of Pediatric Gastroenterology and Nutrition. 2016;**62**(1):169-173. DOI: 10.1097/MPG.0000000000000919

[39] Tume LN, Valla FV. A review of feeding intolerance in critically ill children. European Journal of Pediatrics. 2018;**177**(11):1675-1683. DOI: 10.1007/s00431-018-3229-4

[40] Zafra MA, Molina F, Puerto A. The neural/cephalic phase reflexes in the physiology of nutrition. Neuroscience and Biobehavioral Reviews. 2006;**30**(7):1032-1044. DOI: 10.1016/j.neubiorev.2006.03.005

[41] Zafra MA, Molina F, Puerto A. Rewarding effects of cephalic nutrients and the vagal-brain axis. In: Zafra MA, Molina F, Puerto A, editors. The Cephalic/Neural Phase in Nutrition. Kerala: Research Signpost; 2009. pp. 117-147

[42] Pavlov I. The Work of the Digestive Glands. London: Charles Griffin & Co; 1910

[43] Wood JD. The first Nobel prize for integrated systems physiology: Ivan Petrovich Pavlov, 1904. Physiology (Bethesda, Md.). 2004;**19**:326-330. DOI: 10.1152/physiol.00034.2004

[44] Zafra MA, Molina F, Puerto A. The cephalic/neural phase of digestion: Historical perspective. In: Zafra MΛ, Molina F, Puerto A, editors. The Cephalic/Neural Phase in Nutrition. Kerala: Research Signpost; 2009. pp. 1-32

[45] Oades RD, Halliday GM. Ventral tegmental (A10) system: Neurobiology. 1. Anatomy and connectivity. Brain Research. 1987;**434**(2):117-165. DOI: 10.1016/0165-0173(87)90011-7

[46] Love JA, Yi E, Smith TG. Autonomic pathways regulating pancreatic exocrine secretion. Autonomic Neuroscience. 2007;**133**(1):19-34. DOI: 10.1016/j.autneu.2006.10.001

[47] Li CS, Lu DP, Cho YK. Descending projections from the nucleus accumbens

shell excite activity of taste-responsive neurons in the nucleus of the solitary tract in the hamster. Journal of Neurophysiology. 2015;**113**(10):3778-3786. DOI: 10.1152/jn.00362.2014

[48] Carey MC, Small DM, Bliss CM. Lipid digestion and absorption. Annual Review of Physiology. 1983;**45**:651-677. DOI: 10.1146/annurev.ph.45.030183.003251

[49] Giduck SA, Threatte RM, Kare MR. Cephalic reflexes: Their role in digestion and possible roles in absorption and metabolism. The Journal of Nutrition. 1987;**117**(7):1191-1196. DOI: 10.1093/jn/117.7.1191

[50] Kulkarni BV, Mattes RD. Lingual lipase activity in the orosensory detection of fat by humans. American Journal of Physiology. Regulatory, Integrative and Comparative Physiology. 2014;**306**(12):R879-R885. DOI: 10.1152/ajpregu.00352.2013

[51] Kemmer T, Malfertheiner P. Influence of atropine on taste-stimulated parotid secretion. Research in Experimental Medicine (Berlin). 1985;**185**(6):495-502. DOI: 10.1007/BF01851855

[52] Konturek SJ, Konturek JW. Cephalic phase of pancreatic secretion. Appetite. 2000;**34**(2):197-205. DOI: 10.1006/appe.1999.0281

[53] Hiraoka T, Fukuwatari T, Imaizumi M, Fushiki T. Effects of oral stimulation with fats on the cephalic phase of pancreatic enzyme secretion in esophagostomized rats. Physiology & Behavior. 2003;**79**(4-5):713-717. DOI: 10.1016/S0031-9384(03)00201-4

[54] Mattes RD. Oral fatty acid signaling and intestinal lipid processing: Support and supposition. Physiology & Behavior. 2011;**105**(1):27-35. DOI: 10.1016/j.physbeh.2011.02.016

[55] Kokrashvili Z, Yee KK, Ilegems E, Iwatsuki K, Li Y, Mosinger B, et al. Endocrine taste cells. The British Journal of Nutrition. 2014;**111**(Suppl 1):S23-S29. DOI: 10.1017/S0007114513002262

[56] Zhu Y, Hsu WH, Hollis JH. Modified sham feeding of foods with different macronutrient compositions differentially influences cephalic change of insulin, ghrelin, and NMR-based metabolomic profiles. Physiology & Behavior. 2014;**135**:135-142. DOI: 10.1016/j.physbeh.2014.06.009

[57] Robertson MD. Food perception and postprandial lipid metabolism. Physiology & Behavior. 2006;**89**(1):4-9. DOI: 10.1016/j.physbeh.2006.01.030

[58] Stern RM, Crawford HE, Stewart WR, Vasey MW, Koch KL. Sham feeding. Cephalic-vagal influences on gastric myoelectric activity. Digestive Diseases and Sciences. 1989;**34**(4):521-527. DOI: 10.1007/BF01536327

[59] Katschinski M, Dahmen G, Reinshagen M, Beglinger C, Koop H, Nustede R, et al. Cephalic stimulation of gastrointestinal secretory and motor responses in humans. Gastroenterology. 1992;**103**(2):383-391. DOI: 10.1016/0016-5085(92)90825-J

[60] Chen JD, Pan J, Orr WC. Role of sham feeding in postprandial changes of gastric myoelectrical activity. Digestive Diseases and Sciences. 1996;**41**(9):1706-1712. DOI: 10.1007/BF02088734

[61] Waluga M, Jonderko K, Domosławska E, Matwiejszyn A, Dzielicki M, Krusiec-Świdergoł B, et al. Effects of taste stimulation on gastric myoelectrical activity and autonomic balance. Saudi Journal of Gastroenterology. 2018;**24**(2):100-108. DOI: 10.4103/sjg.SJG_419_17

[62] Molina F, Thiel T, Deutsch JA, Puerto A. Comparison between some digestive processes after

eating and gastric loading in rats. Pharmacology, Biochemistry, and Behavior. 1977;7(4):347-350. DOI: 10.1016/0091-3057(77)90230-1

[63] Friedman MI, Ramirez I, Tordoff MG. Gastric emptying of ingested fat emulsion in rats: Implications for studies of fat-induced satiety. The American Journal of Physiology. 1996;**270**(3 Pt 2): R688-R692. DOI: 10.1152/ajpregu.1996.270.3.R688

[64] Morey S, Shafat A, Clegg ME. Oral versus intubated feeding and the effect on glycaemic and insulinaemic responses, gastric emptying and satiety. Appetite. 2016;**96**:598-603. DOI: 10.1016/j.appet.2015.11.002

[65] Snowdon CT. Gastrointestinal sensory and motor control of food intake. Journal of Comparative and Physiological Psychology. 1970;**71**(1):68-76. DOI: 10.1037/h0028964

[66] Ramirez I, Tordoff MG, Friedman MI. Satiety from fat? Adverse effects of intestinal infusion of sodium oleate. The American Journal of Physiology. 1997;**273**(5 Pt 2):R1779-R1785. DOI: 10.1152/ajpregu.1997.273.5.R1779

[67] Proietto J, Rohner-Jeanrenaud F, Ionescu E, Jeanrenaud B. Role of the oropharynx in regulation of glycemia. Diabetes. 1987;**36**(7):791-795. DOI: 10.2337/diab.36.7.791

[68] Storlien LH, Bruce DG. Mind over metabolism: The cephalic phase in relation to non-insulin-dependent diabetes and obesity. Biological Psychology. 1989;**28**(1):3-23. DOI: 10.1016/0301-0511(89)90108-7

[69] Mennella I, Ferracane R, Zucco F, Fogliano V, Vitaglione P. Food liking enhances the plasma response of 2-arachidonoylglycerol and of pancreatic polypeptide upon modified sham feeding in humans. The Journal of Nutrition. 2015;**145**(9):2169-2175. DOI: 10.3945/jn.114.207704

[70] Brede S, Sputh A, Hartmann AC, Hallschmid M, Lehnert H, Klement J. Visual food cues decrease postprandial glucose concentrations in lean and obese men without affecting food intake and related endocrine parameters. Appetite. 2017;**117**:255-262. DOI: 10.1016/j.appet.2017.07.001

[71] Teff KL, Engelman K. Oral sensory stimulation improves glucose tolerance in humans: Effects on insulin, C-peptide, and glucagon. The American Journal of Physiology. 1996;**270**(6 Pt 2):R1371-R1379. DOI: 10.1152/ajpregu.1996.270.6.R1371

[72] McGregor IS, Lee AM. Changes in respiratory quotient elicited in rats by a conditioned stimulus predicting food. Physiology & Behavior. 1998;**63**(2):227-232. DOI: 10.1016/S0031-9384(97)00429-0

[73] Kamath MV, Spaziani R, Ullal S, Tougas G, Guzman JC, Morillo C, et al. The effect of sham feeding on neurocardiac regulation in healthy human volunteers. Canadian Journal of Gastroenterology. 2007;**21**(11):721-726. DOI: 10.1155/2007/891374

[74] Deighton K, Duckworth L, Matu J, Suter M, Fletcher C, Stead S, et al. Mouth rinsing with a sweet solution increases energy expenditure and decreases appetite during 60 min of self-regulated walking exercise. Applied Physiology, Nutrition, and Metabolism. 2016;**41**(12):1255-1261. DOI: 10.1139/apnm-2016-0344

[75] Eguchi K, Kashima H, Yokota A, Miura K, Yamaoka Endo M, Hirano H, et al. Acute effect of oral sensation of sweetness on celiac artery blood flow and gastric myoelectrical activity in humans. Autonomic Neuroscience: Basic and Clinical. 2016;**197**:41-45. DOI: 10.1016/j.autneu.2016.03.002

[76] Drazen DL, Vahl TP, D'Alessio DA, Seeley RJ, Woods SC. Effects of a fixed meal pattern on ghrelin secretion: Evidence for a learned response independent of nutrient status. Endocrinology. 2006;**147**(1):23-30. DOI: 10.1210/en.2005-0973

[77] Monteleone P, Serritella C, Scognamiglio P, Maj M. Enhanced ghrelin secretion in the cephalic phase of food ingestion in women with bulimia nervosa. Psychoneuroendocrinology. 2010;**35**(2):284-828. DOI: 10.1016/j.psyneuen.2009.07.001

[78] Madhu V, Shirali A, Pawaskar PN, Madi D, Chowta N, Ramapuram JT. Mastication frequency and postprandial blood sugar levels in normoglycaemic and dysglycaemic individuals: A cross- sectional comparative study. Journal of Clinical and Diagnostic Research. 2016;**10**(7):OC06-OOC8. DOI: 10.7860/JCDR/2016/18855.8082

[79] Glendinning JI, Lubitz GS, Shelling S. Taste of glucose elicits cephalic-phase insulin release in mice. Physiology & Behavior. 2018;**192**:200-205. DOI: 10.1016/j.physbeh.2018.04.002

[80] Puerto A, Deutsch JA, Molina F, Roll PL. Rapid discrimination of rewarding nutrient by the upper gastrointestinal tract. Science. 1976;**192**(4238):485-487. DOI: 10.1126/science.1257784

[81] Zafra MA, Simón MJ, Molina F, Puerto A. The role of the external lateral parabrachial subnucleus in flavor preferences induced by predigested food administered intragastrically. Brain Research. 2002;**950**(1-2):155-164. DOI: 10.1016/S0006-8993(02)03032-9

[82] Mediavilla C, Mahía J, Bernal A, Puerto A. The D2/D3-receptor antagonist tiapride impairs concurrent but not sequential taste aversion learning. Brain Research Bulletin. 2012;**87**(2-3):346-349. DOI: 10.1016/j.brainresbull.2011.10.022

[83] Zafra MA, Prados M, Molina F, Puerto A. Capsaicin-sensitive afferent vagal fibers are involved in concurrent taste aversion learning. Neurobiology of Learning and Memory. 2006;**86**(3):349-352. DOI: 10.1016/j.nlm.2006.07.004

[84] Deutsch JA, Molina F, Puerto A. Conditioned taste aversion caused by palatable nontoxic nutrients. Behavioral Biology. 1976;**16**(2):161-174. DOI: 10.1016/S0091-6773(76)91268-2

[85] Zafra MA, Simón MJ, Molina F, Puerto A. Lesions of the lateral parabrachial area block the aversive component and induced-flavor preference for the delayed intragastric administration of nutrients in rats: Effects on subsequent food and water intake. Nutritional Neuroscience. 2005;**8**(5-6):297-307. DOI: 10.1080/10284150600576655

[86] Zafra MA, Simón MJ, Molina F, Puerto A. Effects of intragastric administration of predigested nutrients on food intake, body weight and taste acceptability: Potential relevance of the cephalic/neural phase of digestion. Nutritional Neuroscience. 2007;**10**(1-2):97-103. DOI: 10.1016/S0006-8993(02)03032-9

[87] Zafra MA, Molina F, Puerto A. Learned flavor preferences induced by intragastric administration of rewarding nutrients: role of capsaicin-sensitive vagal afferent fibers. American Journal of Physiology. Regulatory, Integrative and Comparative Physiology. 2007;**293**(2):R635-R641. DOI: 10.1152/ajpregu.00136.2007

[88] Zafra MA, Agüera AD, Molina F, Puerto A. Relevance of the nucleus of the solitary tract, gelatinous part, in learned preferences induced by intragastric nutrient administration. Appetite. 2017;**118**:90-96. DOI: 10.1016/j.appet.2017.08.004

[89] Wolf S. The psyche and the stomach. A historical vignette. Gastroenterology. 1981;**80**(3):605-614

[90] Wolf S, Wolff HG. Human Gastric Function. An Experimental Study of a Man and his Stomach. London: Oxford University Press; 1947. 262 p

[91] Janowitz HD, Hollander F, Orringer D, Levy MH, Winkelstein A, Kaufman R, et al. A quantitative study of the gastric secretory response to sham feeding in a human subject. Gastroenterology. 1950;**16**(1):104-116

[92] Parker JG, Werther JL, Hollander F. Gastric cation secretion in a patient with complete esophageal obstruction and permanent gastrotomy. Digestive Diseases and Sciences. 1963;**8**(4):319-329. DOI: 10.1007/BF02237704

[93] Yamamoto S, Tomoe M, Toyama K, Kawai M, Uneyama H. Can dietary supplementation of monosodium glutamate improve the health of the elderly? The American Journal of Clinical Nutrition. 2009;**90**(3):844S-849S. DOI: 10.3945/ajcn.2009.27462X

[94] Sasano T, Satoh-Kuriwada S, Shoji N, Iikubo M, Kawai M, Uneyama H, et al. Important role of umami taste sensitivity in oral and overall health. Current Pharmaceutical Design. 2014;**20**(16):2750-2754. DOI: 10.2174/13816128113199990577

[95] Potana NT, Dongara AR, Nimbalkar SM, Patel DV, Nimbalkar AS, Phatak A. Oral sucrose for pain in neonates during echocardiography: a randomized controlled trial. Indian Pediatriatrics. 2015;**52**(6):493-497

[96] Crystal SR, Teff KL. Tasting fats: Cephalic phase hormonal responses and food intake in restrained and unrestrained eaters. Physiology and Behavior. 2006;**89**(2):213-220. DOI: 10.1016/j.physbeh.2006.06.013

[97] Sengupta JN, Gebhart GF. In: Johnson LR, editor. Physiology of the gastrointestinal tractGastrointestinal Afferent Fibers and Sensation. New York: Raven Press; 1994. pp. 483-519

[98] Novin D. The integration of visceral information in the control of feeding. Journal of the Autonomic Nervous System. 1983;**9**(1):233-246. DOI: 10.1016/0165-1838(83)90144-3

[99] Grundy D. Sensory signals from the gastrointestinal tract. Journal of Pediatric Gastroenterology and Nutrition. 2005;**41**(Suppl 1):S7-S9. DOI: 10.1097/01.scs.0000180286.58988.cf

[100] Zhu JX, Zhu XY, Owyang C, Li Y. Intestinal serotonin acts as a paracrine substance to mediate vagal signal transmission evoked by luminal factors in the rat. The Journal of Physiology. 2001;**530**(Pt 3:431-442. DOI: 10.1111/j.1469-7793.2001.0431k.x

[101] Powley TL, Spaulding RA, Haglof SA. Vagal afferent innervation of the proximal gastrointestinal tract mucosa: Chemoreceptor and mechanoreceptor architecture. The Journal of Comparative Neurology. 2011;**519**(4):644-660. DOI: 10.1002/cne.22541

[102] Dockray GJ. Enteroendocrine cell signaling via the vagus nerve. Current Opinion in Pharmacology. 2013;**13**:954-958. DOI: 10.1016/j.coph.2013.09.007

[103] Janssen S, Depoortere I. Nutrient sensing in the gut: New roads to therapeutics? Trends in Endocrinology and Metabolism. 2013;**24**(2):92-100. DOI: 10.1016/j.tem.2012.11.006

[104] De Lartigue G, Diepenbroek C. Novel developments in vagal afferent nutrient sensing and its role in energy homeostasis. Current Opinion in Pharmacology. 2016;**31**:38-43. DOI: 10.1016/j.coph.2016.08.007

[105] Altschuler SM, Bao XM, Bieger D, Hopkins DA, Miselis RR. Viscerotopic representation of the upper alimentary tract in the rat: Sensory ganglia and nuclei of the solitary and spinal trigeminal tracts. The Journal of Comparative Neurology. 1989;**283**(2):248-268. DOI: 10.1002/cne.902830207

[106] Barraco R, el-Ridi M, Ergene E, Parizon M, Bradley D. An atlas of the rat subpostremal nucleus tractus solitarius. Brain Research Bulletin. 1992;**29**(6):703-765. DOI: 10.1016/0361-9230(92)90143-L

[107] Herbert H, Moga MM, Saper CB. Connections of the parabrachial nucleus with the nucleus of the solitary tract and the medullary reticular formation in the rat. The Journal of Comparative Neurology. 1990;**293**(4):540-580. DOI: 10.1002/cne.902930404

[108] Holzer P. Capsaicin: Cellular targets, mechanisms of action, and selectivity for thin sensory neurons. Pharmacological Reviews. 1991;**43**(2):143-201

[109] Prechtl JC, Powley TP. The fiber composition of the abdominal vagus of the rat. Anatomy and Embryology. 1990;**181**:101-115. DOI: 10.1007/BF00198950

[110] Berthoud HR, Neuhuber WL. Distribution and morphology of vagal afferents supplying the digestive system. In: Taché Y, Wiggate DL, Burks TF, editors. Innervation of the Gut: Pathophysiological Implications. Boca Raton: CRC; 1994. pp. 43-66

[111] Shapiro RE, Miselis RR. The central neural connections of the area postrema of the rat. The Journal of Comparative Neurology. 1985;**234**(3):344-364. DOI: 10.1002/cne.902340306

[112] Fraser KA, Davison JS. Meal-induced c-fos expression in brain stem is not dependent on cholecystokinin release. The American Journal of Physiology. 1993;**265**(1Pt 2):R235-R239. DOI: 10.1152/ajpregu.1993.265.1.R235

[113] Zittel TT, De Giorgio R, Sternini C, Raybould HE. Fos protein expression in the nucleus of the solitary tract in response to intestinal nutrients in awake rats. Brain Research. 1994;**663**(2):266-270. DOI: 10.1016/0006-8993(94)91272-6

[114] Yamamoto T, Sawa K. c-Fos-like immunoreactivity in the brainstem following gastric loads of various chemical solutions in rats. Brain Research. 2000;**866**(1-2):135-143. DOI: 10.1016/S0006-8993(00)02241-1

[115] Emond M, Schwartz GJ, Moran TH. Meal-related stimuli differentially induce c-Fos activation in the nucleus of the solitary tract. American journal of physiology regulatory integrative and comparative. Physiology. 2001;**280**(5):R1315-RR121. DOI: 10.1152/ajpregu.2001.280.5.R1315

[116] Olson BR, Freilino M, Hoffman GE, Stricker EM, Sved AF, Verbalis JG. c-Fos expression in rat brain and brainstem nuclei in response to treatments that alter food intake and gastric motility. Molecular and Cellular Neurosciences. 1993;**4**(1):93-106. DOI: 10.1006/mcne.1993.1011

[117] Zhang X, Fogel R, Renehan WE. Physiology and morphology of neurons in the dorsal motor nucleus of the vagus and the nucleus of the solitary tract that are sensitive to distension of the small intestine. The Journal of Comparative Neurology. 1992;**323**(3):432-448. DOI: 10.1002/cne.903230310

[118] van de Wall EH, Duffy P, Ritter RC. CCK enhances response to gastric distension by acting on capsaicin-sensitive vagal afferents. American Journal of Physiology. Regulatory,

Integrative and Comparative Physiology. 2005;**289**(3):R695-R703. DOI: 10.1152/ajpregu.00809.2004

[119] Young RL, Cooper NJ, Blackshaw LA. Chemical coding and central projections of gastric vagal afferent neurons. Neurogastroenterology and Motility. 2008;**20**(6):708-718. DOI: 10.1111/j.1365-2982.2007.01071.x

[120] Torrealba F, Calderón F. Central projections of coarse and fine vagal axons of the cat. Brain Research. 1990;**510**(2):351-354. DOI: 10.1016/0006-8993(90)91390-3

[121] Jancsó G, Király E. Distribution of chemosensitive primary sensory afferents in the central nervous system of the rat. The Journal of Comparative Neurology. 1980;**190**(4):781-792. DOI: 10.1002/cne.901900409

[122] Fulwiler CE, Saper CB. Subnuclear organization of the efferent connections of the parabrachial nucleus in the rat. Brain Research Reviews. 1984;**7**(3):229-259. DOI: 10.1016/0165-0173(84)90012-2

[123] Acuña-Goycolea C, Fuentealba P, Torrealba F. Anatomical substrate for separate processing of ascending and descending visceral information in the nucleus of the solitary tract of the rat. Brain Research. 2000;**883**(2):229-232. DOI: 10.1016/S0006-8993(00)02845-6

[124] Gieroba ZJ, Blessing WW. Fos-containing neurons in medulla and pons after unilateral stimulation of the afferent abdominal vagus in conscious rabbits. Neuroscience. 1994;**59**(4):851-858. DOI: 10.1016/0306-4522(94)90289-5

[125] Wang L, Cardin S, Martínez V, Taché Y, Lloyd KC. Duodenal loading with glucose induces fos expression in rat brain: Selective blockade by devazepide. The American Journal of Physiology. 1999;**277**(3 Pt 2):R667-R674. DOI: 10.1152/ajpregu.1999.277.3.R667.

[126] Li BH, Rowland NE. Effects of vagotomy on cholecystokinin- and dexfenfluramine-induced Fos-like immunoreactivity in the rat brain. Brain Research Bulletin. 1995;**37**(6):589-593. DOI: 10.1016/0361-9230(95)00045-G

[127] Li BH, Rowland NE. Peripherally and centrally administered bombesin induce Fos-like immunoreactivity in different brain regions in rats. Regulatory Peptides. 1996;**62**(2-3):167-172. DOI: 10.1016/0167-0115(96)00029-8

[128] Horn CC, Friedman MI. 2,5-Anhydro-D-mannitol induces Fos-like immunoreactivity in hindbrain and forebrain: Relationship to eating behavior. Brain Research. 1998;**779**(1-2):17-25. DOI: 10.1016/S0006-8993(97)01073-1

[129] Horn CC, Friedman MI. Methyl palmoxirate increases eating behavior and brain Fos-like immunoreactivity in rats. Brain Research. 1998;**781**(1-2):8-14. DOI: 10.1016/S0006-8993(97)01143-8

[130] Horn CC, Tordoff MG, Friedman MI. Role of vagal afferent innervation in feeding and brain Fos expression produced by metabolic inhibitors. Brain Research. 2001;**919**(2):198-206. DOI: 10.1016/S0006-8993(01)02963-8

[131] Yang H, Wang L, Wu SV, Tay J, Goulet M, Boismenu R, et al. Peripheral secretin-induced Fos expression in the rat brain is largely vagal dependent. Neuroscience. 2004;**128**(1):131-141. DOI: 10.1016/j.neuroscience.2004.06.027

[132] Smith GP, Jerome C, Cushin BJ, Eterno R, Simansky KJ. Abdominal vagotomy blocks the satiety effect of cholecystokinin in the rat. Science. 1981;**213**(4511):1036-1037. DOI: 10.1126/science.7268408

[133] Ladenheim EE, Ritter RC. Capsaicin attenuates bombesin-induced suppression of food intake.

The American Journal of Physiology. 1991;**260**(2 Pt 2):R263-R266. DOI: 10.1152/ajpregu.1991.260.2.R263

[134] Ritter S, Dinh TT, Friedman MI. Induction of Fos-like immunoreactivity (Fos-li) and stimulation of feeding by 2,5-anhydro-D-mannitol (2,5-AM) require the vagus nerve. Brain Research. 1994;**646**(1):53-64. DOI: 10.1016/0006-8993(94)90057-4

[135] Simon MJ, Garcia R, Zafra MA, Molina F, Puerto A. Learned preferences induced by electrical stimulation of a food-related area of the parabrachial complex: Effects of naloxone. Neurobiology of Learning and Memory. 2007;**87**(3):332-342. DOI: 10.1016/j.nlm.2006.09.009

[136] Zafra MA, Molina F, Puerto A. Chemical afferent vagal axotomy blocks re-intake after partial withdrawal of gastric food contents. Nutritional Neuroscience. 2017;**20**(10):587-597. DOI: 10.1080/1028415X.2016.1208970

[137] Zafra MA, Agüera AD, Molina F, Puerto A. Disruption of re-intake after partial withdrawal of gastric food contents in rats lesioned in the gelatinous part of the nucleus of the solitary tract. Appetite. 2017;**113**:231-238. DOI: 10.1016/j.appet.2017.02.040

[138] Zafra MA, Agüera AD, Simón MJ, Molina F, Puerto A. Satiation and re-intake after partial withdrawal of gastric food contents: A dissociation effect in external lateral parabrachial lesioned rats. Brain Research Bulletin. 2016;**127**:126-133. DOI: 10.1016/j.brainresbull.2016.09.006

[139] Mediavilla C, Bernal A, Mahía J, Puerto A. Nucleus of the solitary tract and flavor aversion learning: Relevance in concurrent but not sequential behavioral test. Behavioural Brain Research. 2011;**223**(2):287-292. DOI: 10.1016/j.bbr.2011.04.044

[140] Mediavilla C, Molina F, Puerto A. The role of the lateral parabrachial nuclei in concurrent and sequential taste aversion learning in rats. Experimental Brain Research. 2000;**134**(4):497-505. DOI: 10.1007/s002210000497